the mothercare guide to
EMERGENCIES
— AND —
FIRST AID

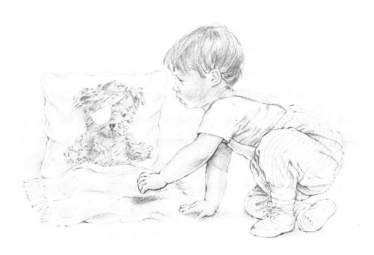

in association with
THE BRITISH RED CROSS SOCIETY

Anne Davies

Conran Octopus

Project editor	Jane O'Shea
Editor	Emma Russell
Project assistant	Debora Robertson
Art editor	Prue Bucknall
Production	Shane Lask
Illustrations	Lucy Su
Jacket photograph	Andy Cox

First published in 1989 by
Conran Octopus Limited
37 Shelton Street
London WC2H 9HN

ISBN 1 85029 165 9

Typeset by Bookworm Typesetting, Manchester
Printed by Eagle Press plc, Scotland

CONTENTS

INTRODUCTION

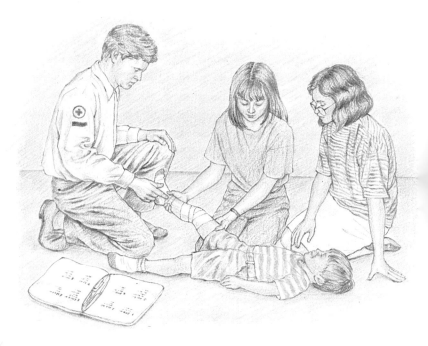

Would you know what to do if your child poured a cup of hot tea over himself, fell downstairs and knocked himself out, or cut himself on a sharp knife and had blood spurting from his arm?

Preventing such accidents is obviously preferable to them happening. But children are particularly vulnerable to accidents and, however careful you are, your child will almost certainly experience some injuries and may be unlucky enough to suffer a serious accident. This book gives you the information you need to cope with situations ranging from major emergencies that may threaten your child's life to minor scrapes and bangs.

The first two chapters offer advice on being prepared for an emergency, taking steps to prevent accidents happening in the first place and coping with an emergency situation. Chapter three describes how to carry out the most important emergency techniques – for maintaining breathing, restoring heart beat, controlling bleeding and dealing with unconsciousness and shock. The information given in this chapter is central to the whole book and it has therefore been printed on tinted pages for easy reference. Chapter four gives step-by-step instructions for treatment in emergencies. The final chapters provide a suggested list of first aid equipment, guidance on how to put on dressings, bandages and slings, and an A-Z of treatments for common childhood injuries.

When treating children, bear in mind that the size of a child affects the rate of his breathing and heartbeat; the smaller the child, the faster the rate. His size also affects the way you carry out some first aid treatments, such as mouth-to-mouth ventilation, external chest compression and dealing with choking. These need to be done slightly differently on a young child or baby and, where this is the case, the differences are clearly described and illustrated.

It is a good idea to familiarize yourself with the techniques described here before you find yourself in a situation where you need to use them. The best way to do this is to attend a first aid course such as those run by the British Red Cross Society, St John Ambulance or St Andrew's Ambulance Association (for Scotland) – see page 62 for addresses. The most important life-saving techniques are mouth-to-mouth ventilation (the kiss of life) and cardio-pulmonary resuscitation (external chest compression done in conjunction with mouth-to-mouth ventilation). The first aid organizations recommend that you do not carry out these techniques until you have received proper training from a qualified instructor.

If your child goes to a playgroup or nursery, or if you belong to an organization such as the National Childbirth Trust, see if you can persuade them to organize a course on first aid for babies and small children for you and other parents.

If your child is hurt or in pain, remember to comfort and reassure him as well as giving him first aid. Try not to forget this while you are coping with the accident and don't leave him unless you have to. If you can stay calm, this will help your child to feel secure and less frightened and will also help you think through what you need to do.

You will find that the sections on dealing with specific situations frequently end with advice to seek medical help from a doctor or hospital casualty department. If you have *any* doubts about the nature or extent of your child's injuries, you should seek medical advice; it is always best to be on the safe side.

REMEMBER

When treating a child, keep in mind the principles of first aid:
> ▶ to preserve the child's life
> ▶ to prevent any deterioration in his condition
> ▶ to promote his recovery.

This book is one of a series of Mothercare Guides that covers topics of immediate interest to parents of young children. The books are all fully illustrated and offer clear and straightforward guidance on practical aspects of everyday childcare. The other titles available in the series are listed on the back jacket of this book.

All the information in these books applies equally to male and female children. To reflect this, the pronouns 'he' and 'she' have been used in alternating chapters throughout each book. Where, occasionally, the text does apply to a particular sex, the appropriate pronoun is used.

BEING PREPARED

You will feel more confident in being able to cope with an accident, whether major or minor, if you know you are as well prepared as possible. Keep a first aid box at home and make sure it is kept well stocked (see pages 52–3 for what you need in it). Carry a smaller one in the car that you can also take on holiday.

Write down the address, phone number and opening times of your nearest hospital accident and emergency (casualty) department. Don't forget to record the same details for your family doctor; keep this information by the phone and ensure that anyone looking after your child knows that it is there. If you have a car, work out the route from your house to the hospital and drive it, so you'll know exactly where to go when you need to – it could save valuable time one day.

ACCIDENT PREVENTION AND SAFETY

Up to about twenty per cent of small children have to visit a hospital accident and emergency department each year. In many of these cases, no actual treatment is required, but around 800 children in England and Wales die each year after an accident. Falls are the most frequent non-fatal injury amongst the under-fours, although burns cause most deaths. In children aged five and over, most accidents are outside the home, with road accidents posing the greatest threat.

There are several steps you can take to minimize the risk of accidents happening to your child, and the time you spend in thinking about potential hazards and taking appropriate precautions may spare your child – and you – from much unnecessary pain and distress.

Teach your child, from a young age, the basic rules of road safety and make her aware of the dangers as well as the fun of water. At home, check that gates and doors are secured and fences mended,

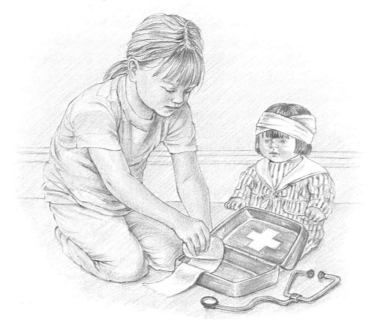

AUTHORIZATION FOR EMERGENCY TREATMENT

Permission from parents is necessary before a child can receive certain treatments, such as stitching, an anaesthetic or a blood transfusion. If your child is looked after regularly by, for example, a grandparent, childminder or nanny, it would be sensible to give them a letter, signed by both parents, permitting them to authorize doctors to carry out treatment in an emergency. This could save precious time if your child's life is at risk and you are not easily contactable.

so there is no danger of her running out into the street unsupervised. Never leave her alone near water, whether in the house or outside. Babies and young children don't understand about holding their breath – their automatic reflex is to breathe in and this is why they can drown so easily. It is a good idea to teach your child to swim from a young age and many babies really enjoy it. Local swimming baths often run swimming classes for children. Another sensible precaution is for you to learn to swim properly. If you are a good swimmer yourself, you will be able to give your child confidence in learning to swim and will also be in a better position to help her if she gets into difficulty in the water. You might also consider taking a course in life saving, such as the ones run by the Royal Life Saving Society (see page 62 for address).

Very young babies may suffocate in their cot if they have a pillow so don't use one until your baby is at least a year old. Don't let a baby play with anything small enough to go in her mouth or leave her alone with a bottle or any other food – she could easily choke in your absence.

Falls are a major cause of accidents in the home. Secure rugs and mats so they cannot slip; make sure that there are no toys lying about to be tripped over; and never leave a flex trailing where anyone could catch their foot in it (or where a child could pull whatever it is attached to down on her head).

As soon as your baby can move independently – even just rolling – falls are a hazard. Even if you use a stair gate, teach your baby how to climb up and down stairs safely as soon as she starts to explore them. Older babies often wriggle a lot when their nappy is being changed so never leave them unattended on a raised surface. Always use a separate safety harness in highchairs, pushchairs and prams.

Poisoning is another danger – young children tend to put everything in their mouths. Keep items like bleach, medicines, oven cleaner, insecticides and disinfectant locked away or well out of reach. Many common garden plants are dangerous when eaten so supervise very small children and teach older ones not to eat anything from the garden.

Burns and scalds are most likely to occur in the kitchen. Keep hot drinks, teapots and kettles well out of reach. Use a guard on the cooker and keep your child away from it while you are cooking; splashes of hot fat or liquid could land on her. Preferably, keep her out of the kitchen altogether.

Always use a guard round fires (gas and electric, as well as open) and watch that radiators and pipes don't get too hot. Turn down the thermostat on your hot water system, so the hot water is not scalding when it comes out of the tap. Unplug electrical appliances when you are not using them and cover unused sockets with socket covers.

COPING IN AN EMERGENCY

If you are faced with an emergency – your child is unconscious, badly burnt or bleeding severely – the most important thing is to stay calm. Take a deep breath and try not to panic while you think what action to take. If you remain calm, it will also help to reassure your child. The best way of dealing with an emergency is by:

- ▶ making a quick assessment of the situation and the injured child
- ▶ working out what has happened, from what you can see, what the injured child or anyone else can tell you and from the child's injuries or symptoms
- ▶ giving immediate and appropriate treatment for any injuries.

Use your common sense and do not attempt to do too much. If you are in any doubt about the extent of your child's injuries, call for medical help immediately.

APPROACH

- ▶ Make a quick assessment of the situation to check whether there is either a risk of danger to yourself or of further injury to anyone involved (see Hazardous situations, pages 12–13).
- ▶ If more than one child has been hurt, treat the most severely injured first. Always remember that the child who is crying loudest may not necessarily be the one who has the most serious injuries.
- ▶ Try and find out what is wrong; if he is conscious, ask the child how he feels. Find out, for example, if he hurts anywhere or can't move a limb. Check his rate of breathing (this should normally be 20–30 breaths a minute) and his pulse rate (normally 80–100 beats a minute).
- ▶ If a child is unconscious, check the 'ABC' priorities – Airway, Breathing and Circulation (see pages 10–11). Check for any severe bleeding and control it immediately (see page 22).
- ▶ Place an unconscious child, or one who is breathing noisily, in the recovery position (see page 20), unless you suspect a fracture.
- ▶ If you suspect a fracture (see page 44), don't move him unless you have to, in order to avoid further injury.
- ▶ Shock (see page 23) may develop after a serious accident or injury. Keep your child warm, quiet and lying down until medical help arrives.

ASSESSING INJURIES

After checking your child's airway, breathing and circulation, quickly make a general examination to assess what is wrong. Start at his head and work down. If he is conscious, reassure him as you examine him. These are some general rules to follow:

> ▶ move him as little as possible
> ▶ use all your senses: look, feel, listen and smell
> ▶ compare one side of his body to the other to see if there is any irregularity or swelling.

Look inside his mouth for anything like blood or loose teeth which may cause choking. Look at his lips for signs of burns from corrosive poison. Check his nose and ears for signs of blood or a straw-coloured discharge which may indicate a fractured skull. Run your hands gently over his skull – any bleeding, swelling or indentation may also mean a fracture. Feel his pulse and look at his face. Is the pulse strong but slow? Is his skin dry and flushed? Are his pupils of unequal size? If so, he could have compression of the brain. On the other hand, is his pulse rapid but weak? Is his skin cold and clammy? Is his breathing shallow? Does he seem confused? If so, suspect that he may have concussion.

Moving down from his head, check his collar bone, breastbone and ribcage by gently running your fingers over them. Feel at the hollow of his neck and back for any irregularity of the spine. If you suspect that his spine may be fractured, **do not move him** – call for medical help as soon as possible. Next, check the pelvic area and his arms and legs for deformity, swelling and dampness.

Children suffering from some medical conditions, such as epilepsy or diabetes, may wear a medical warning item round their wrist or neck, so look out for anything like this.

GETTING HELP

If you are at all uncertain about the nature or extent of a child's injuries, get him to the nearest hospital casualty department. If you have a car, take him yourself or, better still, ask a friend to drive while you comfort and reassure the child. In certain situations, however, an ambulance may be necessary to provide trained medical care on the way to the hospital. You should call an ambulance after all serious accidents and any incident which involves:

● difficulty in breathing
● heart failure
● severe bleeding
● unconsciousness
● serious burns
● suspected fracture of the neck or spine
● shock
● poisoning.

If possible, stay with your child and get someone else to phone the emergency services.

To contact the emergency services, dial 999 and ask for the service or services you need – probably ambulance. Give your phone number so that if you are cut off for any reason the switchboard can call you back.

Give precise details of where the casualty is, describing any landmarks which may help the ambulance driver find the site. Also say what has happened, the number and age of those injured, and the extent of the injuries. Don't put the phone down before the ambulance control officer.

ACTION PRIORITIES

Breathing is an essential process if life is to continue. When you breathe, oxygen is taken into the lungs and distributed round the body by the blood; without oxygen, parts of the brain can die after only three minutes. It is most important to maintain breathing and blood circulation in an unconscious child, so check the 'ABC' priorities first and take the appropriate action (see chart below):

A   **AIRWAY** Open your child's airway (see pages 14–15) to allow air into his lungs.

B   **BREATHING** If he has stopped breathing, use mouth-to-mouth ventilation (see pages 16–17) to get air into his lungs.

C   **CIRCULATION** If his heart has stopped, apply external chest compression (see pages 18–19) to pump blood round his body to the vital organs. Control severe bleeding, so blood circulation can continue efficiently.

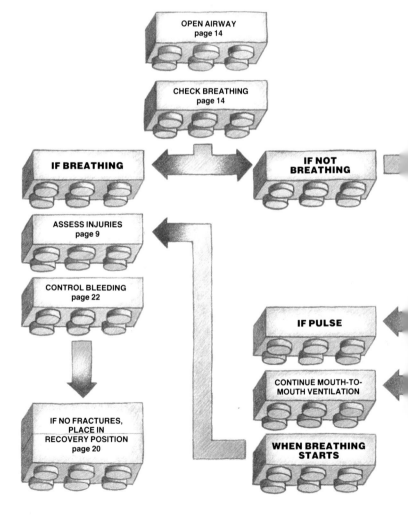

EMERGENCY CHECKLIST

In an emergency, it helps to be aware of the main aim in treating an injury or condition. Use this list as quick reference before turning to the pages indicated for full information on how to treat the situation.

ASPHYXIA: restore breathing, see page 25
BLEEDING: press on source of bleeding, see page 22
BURNS: cool quickly, see pages 32−5
CHOKING: remove obstruction, see pages 36−7
CONVULSIONS: do not restrict movement, see page 39
DROWNING: restore breathing, see page 40
FRACTURE: do not move casualty, see pages 44−7
POISONING: keep casualty calm, see pages 50−1
UNCONSCIOUSNESS: check breathing and circulation, see pages 20−1

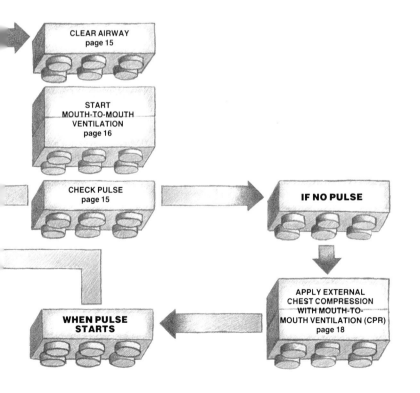

HAZARDOUS SITUATIONS

After certain kinds of accident one of the priorities is to minimize the risk of danger to yourself or other people around and to prevent any further harm coming to your injured child or anyone else hurt in the accident. This might be particularly important after a road accident, in a fire or if your child has been electrocuted, overcome by poisonous fumes or is at risk of drowning.

You must stay calm and make a quick assessment of the situation to decide what to do first. Consider whether you and your child are in any danger; if your child has any life-threatening conditions; if there is anyone around who can help you; and whether you need to call for assistance.

ROAD ACCIDENTS

A high proportion of those injured in serious road accidents are under fourteen years old, so teach your child basic road safety rules.

If you find yourself at the scene of a road accident, first make sure neither you nor anyone injured is in further danger. If a car has crashed, turn off the car engine and don't let anyone smoke near the car. If you can, disconnect the battery. Get someone to warn approaching traffic or use a warning triangle. Send someone to phone the emergency services (see Getting help, page 9).

Don't move anyone who is injured unless it is absolutely necessary (for example, if there is a risk of fire or

danger from oncoming traffic), especially if the injured person is unconscious. Wherever possible, move the danger away from the casualty in preference to moving the casualty. If you do have to move someone, immobilize him as far as possible and try and get enough people to support all parts of his body when you lift him.

Look inside and outside the car for any small children who may have fallen out of sight or been thrown from the vehicle.

If a child is trapped in a vehicle, stay by him and reassure him until medical help arrives. Watch him for signs of shock (see page 23).

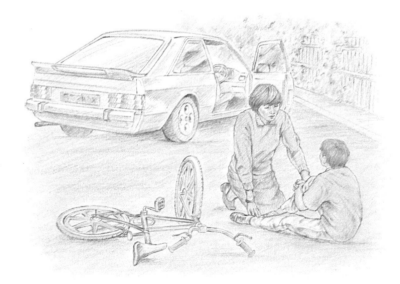

▶ *See pages 32–5 for burns*
▶ *See page 34 for smoke inhalation*

FIRE

Fire spreads quickly. The danger comes not just from flames but also from smoke and toxic fumes – much modern furniture, for example, gives off poisonous fumes which spread very quickly and can kill in just a few seconds.

Contact the emergency services immediately. If the fire is indoors, get everyone out of the building and shut all doors and windows in rooms where it is burning. Don't try to enter a burning room or a building where there is a fire.

Smoke rises, so if you find yourself in a fire, get down on your hands and knees and stay near a window until help arrives. When it does, get any children out first and then follow.

Put out small fires by pouring on water. Don't throw water on a petrol or oil fire: leave it to the fire brigade. With electrical fires, always switch off the power at the mains first and unplug the appliance before trying to put out the flames.

Fires in saucepans can be extinguished by covering them completely with a lid, damp cloth or fire blanket. If something is on fire in an oven, close the oven door and switch it off.

FUMES

Carbon monoxide is a colourless, odourless, poisonous gas; the most common source is car exhaust fumes. If you suspect carbon monoxide poisoning, don't enter the area unless you are sure you are not in any danger and can get out again easily. Take several deep breaths of fresh air before entering and hold your breath while in the gas-filled room or car. Get any casualties into the fresh air for treatment.

Butane and propane gas are used for heating, lighting and refrigerating. Poisoning from these gases should be treated in just the same way as carbon monoxide.

Road accidents may be complicated by the escape of toxic fumes. Most vehicles carrying dangerous substances now display warning signs. If you are in any doubt about the meaning of a sign, keep well away.

DROWNING ACCIDENTS

Do not attempt to rescue a child from deep water or where there is a strong current unless you are a good swimmer. Get help as quickly as possible.

If you can reach the child without endangering your own life, do so. If he has stopped breathing, start mouth-to-mouth ventilation immediately, in the water if necessary. While waiting for an ambulance, keep the child warm. Hypothermia is a possible danger, especially for small children and babies, after even a relatively short time in cold water.

ELECTRICITY

If your child has suffered an electric shock and is still in contact with the electricity, stop the current by switching it off at the mains or pulling out the plug. Don't touch the injured child or even his clothes until this has been done.

If you can't turn off the supply, stand on a dry surface such as a piece of wood, newspaper or a rubber mat and, using a similar material, push the child clear. Don't touch anything wet, as water conducts electricity.

Electricity from overhead cables or electric rails is much more powerful than electricity in the home. Stay at least twenty metres (65 ft) away and call the police. Do not attempt to touch the child or give first aid until you are certain that the power has been switched off.

▶ See page 51 for carbon monoxide poisoning

▶ See page 40 for drowning
▶ See page 41 for electric shock

PRIORITY TECHNIQUES

This chapter contains vital information about treating your child in situations where her life may be at risk, for example if her heart has stopped beating or she is unconscious. Opening her airway and checking her breathing and pulse are essential steps before you apply any other techniques that may be necessary, such as mouth-to-mouth ventilation and external chest compression. Remember the ABC priorities: ensure an open *airway*, restart *breathing* and maintain *circulation*.

OPENING THE AIRWAY

If your child is unconscious, her airway may be narrowed or blocked, making breathing noisy or impossible.

Possible causes for this are:
● the head may be tilted forward, narrowing the air passage
● the tongue may have dropped back, blocking the air passage
● saliva, vomit or other matter may be lying in the back of the throat, blocking the airway.

Any of these situations could lead to your child's death, so you must clear her airway immediately.

▶ If you suspect your child may have spinal injuries (see page 47), **don't** tilt or turn her head – simply pull the lower jaw forward.

1 To open her airway, first kneel beside your child.
2 Lift her chin forward with the index and middle fingers of one hand, while at the same time pressing her forehead back with the heel of your other hand.

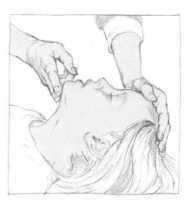

CHECKING BREATHING

Check if your child is breathing by looking, listening and feeling.

1 Continuing to hold your child's airway open, place your ear above her nose and mouth and look along her chest.
2 If your child is breathing, you will see her chest moving and hear and feel the breaths. Place her in the recovery position (see page 20) if she is breathing. If she is not breathing, check her airway is not blocked (see opposite).

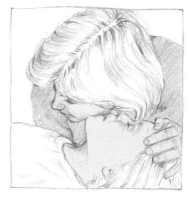

▶ *See page 16 for mouth-to-mouth ventilation*

▶ *See pages 18-19 for external chest compression*

CLEARING THE AIRWAY

Your child's airway may still be blocked after you have opened it, so check for obstructions.

1 Turn your child's head to the side, keeping it well back.

2 Using two fingers, make a quick sweep round the inside of her mouth and lift out any foreign matter.

▶ **Don't** spend time searching for any hidden obstruction and make sure you don't push anything further down your child's throat.

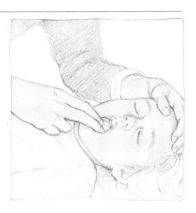

CHECKING THE PULSE

If there is no pulse, your child's heart has stopped beating. You must then immediately begin external chest compression (see pages 18–19) which means pumping the heart artificially. Normal pulse rate for a child is about 80–100 times a minute; the smaller the child, the faster the rate. It can be hard to find the pulse at a time of stress, so practise on your child or even on yourself when you have a quiet moment.

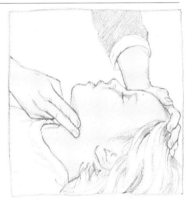

1 Check for a pulse at the child's neck (the carotid pulse). To find the pulse, slide the pads of two or three fingers (not the thumb) across the hollow between her Adam's apple and neck muscle.

2 Keep your fingers there for at least five seconds. If after that time you cannot feel any pulse beating, then the heart can be assumed to have stopped.

FOR A BABY AND YOUNG CHILD

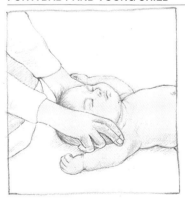

It is sometimes difficult to feel the carotid pulse in a baby or young child. Instead, it is easier to check the brachial pulse which is on the inside of the upper arm, midway between the shoulder and elbow.

1 Place your thumb on the outside of the arm with your index and middle fingers on the inside.

2 Press your fingers lightly towards the bone and feel for at least five seconds.

MOUTH-TO-MOUTH VENTILATION

If your child has stopped breathing, you must use artificial ventilation to get air into her lungs as soon as you can. The most efficient way of doing this is to blow air from your own lungs into hers, by blowing into her mouth – or into the mouth and nose together for babies and young children (see right).

You should always attempt mouth-to-mouth ventilation even if you are in doubt about whether the child can be revived.

It is easiest to give mouth-to-mouth ventilation if the child is lying on her back, but you should start immediately, whatever position she happens to be lying in. The first two inflations must be given slowly. Your child may start breathing again at any stage, but you may still have to use mouth-to-mouth ventilation until breathing settles down to a normal rate. The normal breathing rate for a child is about twenty to thirty times a minute. Don't work too quickly or you will tire yourself out and may begin to feel faint.

Your chances of saving your child's life by applying mouth-to-mouth ventilation will be greatly increased if you have been taught how to do it by a qualified instructor. **Never** practise this technique on a person who is breathing normally.

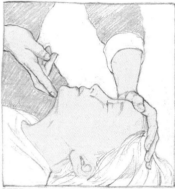 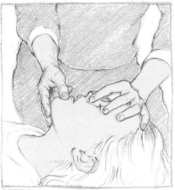

STEP 1

STEP 2

1 Open the child's airway (see page 14) and remove any obstructions or debris you can see in her mouth and throat.

2 Keeping her head well back, with her jaw lifted and mouth open, pinch her nostrils shut with the fingers and thumb of one hand.

3 Take a deep breath, open your mouth wide and seal your lips round the child's mouth. Blow gently but firmly into her mouth; blow in enough air to make her chest rise.

4 Lift your mouth away. Watch your child's chest; you should see it falling as the air comes out.

5 If the chest does not move, check that her head is far enough back and that you have

closed the nostrils properly.

6 Take another deep breath and give your child one more inflation. If there is still no response, your child's airway may be blocked and you must treat for choking (see pages 36–7).

7 After two successful inflations, check the pulse (see page 15) to see if the heart is beating.

If your child's heart is not beating, begin external chest compression immediately (see pages 18–19).

8 If you can feel your child's pulse, and so know her heart is beating, continue giving mouth-to-mouth ventilation about every three seconds (about twenty times a minute). Keep watching her chest while you are

▶ *See page 15 for checking the pulse*

▶ *See pages 18–19 for external chest compression*

FOR A BABY AND YOUNG CHILD

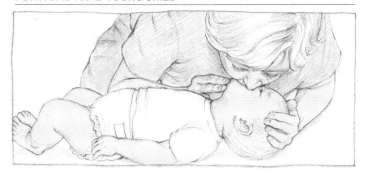

Use mouth-to-mouth-and-nose ventilation for babies and young children. Take care not to tilt a baby's head back too far.

Open the airway. Seal your lips round her mouth and nose and, using gentle puffs, breathe into her lungs at a rate of one breath about every two seconds. Check her pulse after the first two inflations.

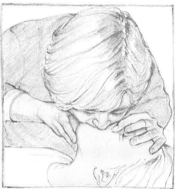

STEP 3

doing this to make sure air is entering her lungs.

9 When your child is breathing independently again, place her in the recovery position (see page 20), but do not leave her alone.

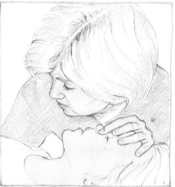

STEP 4

▶ If it is not possible to carry out mouth-to-mouth ventilation, close your child's mouth with your thumb under her lower lip and seal your lips round her nose. Blow gently into her nose. Carry on from step 4 left.

IMPORTANT

▶ Give the first two inflations as soon as possible and in whatever position your child is lying.
▶ Don't spend time looking for hidden obstructions.
▶ Check that her head is tilted back in the correct position: you should be able to see straight down the nostrils.
▶ Make sure that you pinch the soft part of the nostrils shut, not the tip or the bone.
▶ Keep your fingers well clear of your child's mouth so you can form an airtight seal round it with your own mouth.

▶ See page 20 for recovery position

CARDIO-PULMONARY RESUSCITATION

If your child's heart has stopped beating, you must try to restart it as soon as possible. To do this, you apply external chest compression in conjunction with mouth-to-mouth ventilation – this is called cardio-pulmonary resuscitation (CPR). External chest compression involves pressing on the lower half of the breastbone to pump blood out of the heart and round the body, and it must always be preceded and accompanied by mouth-to-mouth ventilation. As soon as you can feel the child's pulse – however faint it is – stop external heart compression immediately, but carry on with mouth-to-mouth if necessary. You should learn how to do CPR from a qualified instructor before attempting this technique on a child. **Never** practise external heart compression on someone whose heart is beating.

EXTERNAL CHEST COMPRESSION

1 Lay your child flat on the ground and kneel beside her, facing her chest. Find the point where the ends of her ribs meet in the middle; this is the bottom of the breastbone.

2 Place the heel of the hand along the line of the breastbone, two finger widths above this middle point. Make sure you keep your fingers off the ribs.

3 Cover your hand with the heel of your other hand and lock your fingers together. Kneel upright so your shoulders are directly over the child's breastbone and your arms are straight.

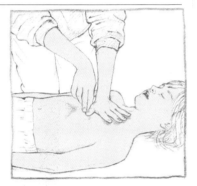

4 Keeping your arms straight, press down about 4–5 centimetres (1½–2 in) then release pressure but do not remove your hands. Do fifteen compressions at a rate of about eighty per minute – find the correct speed by counting 'one-and-two-and . . .' etc. as you work. Compressions should be regular and smooth, not jerky and stabbing.

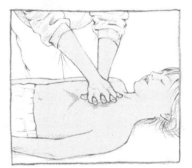

5 After fifteen compressions, move back to your child's head. Tilt your child's head back to re-open her airway and give two more breaths.

6 Continue giving fifteen heart compressions followed by two breaths. Check for the pulse (see page 15) after one minute and then every three minutes.

7 Stop the compressions as soon as your child's pulse returns. Continue with mouth-to-mouth ventilation until she is breathing independently.

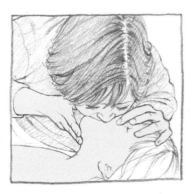

▶ *See page 15 for checking the pulse*

▶ *See pages 16–17 for mouth-to-mouth ventilation*

CPR WITH TWO PEOPLE

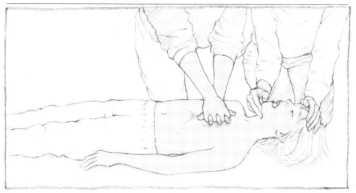

The person at the child's head opens the airway, gives two breaths and checks the pulse. If it is absent, the other person (on the same or opposite side of the child) should begin chest compressions.

The person at the head keeps the airway open and gives a single breath after every fifth compression. Check for the pulse after one minute and then every three minutes.

FOR A YOUNG CHILD

The basic technique is the same as for an older child, but you must work slightly faster and with less pressure. Place the heel of one hand just below the centre of the breastbone (see step 1, opposite). Use light pressure, with one hand only. Press your child's chest at the rate of one hundred compressions a minute and to a depth of 2½–3½ centimetres (1–1½ in). Do five compressions, then one breath, checking for the pulse after one minute, then every three.

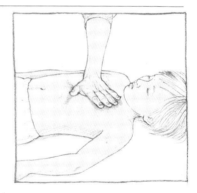

FOR A BABY

For babies and children under two, apply pressure with two fingers only. Make sure the baby is on a firm surface and support her head by sliding one hand behind her neck. Place two fingers just below the centre of the breastbone (see step 1, opposite) and press gently at the rate of one hundred compressions a minute to a depth of 1½–2½ centimetres (½–1 in). Give five compressions to one breath; check for the brachial pulse (see page 15) after one minute, then every three.

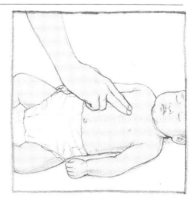

DEALING WITH UNCONSCIOUSNESS

If you find your child unconscious or semi-conscious, your priority must be to keep her airway open and to keep checking whether she is becoming more deeply unconscious (see Checking for response, right). Open your child's airway and check her breathing (see page 14). If necessary, complete the ABC priorities (see pages 16–19).

Once she is breathing, check for signs of serious injury and control any serious bleeding (see page 22). Place her in the recovery position (see below). This keeps the airway open and lets vomit or saliva drain from the mouth without blocking the airway.

Unconsciousness can develop gradually or suddenly, from injury or illness. Common causes include head injury (see page 48); lack of blood supply to the brain, for example, from shock (see page 23); lack of oxygen in the lungs, for example from electrical injury (see page 41), or a blocked airway (see page 14); poisoning (see page 50); diabetes (page 39); heatstroke or hypothermia (see page 49); or epilepsy (see page 41).

RECOVERY POSITION

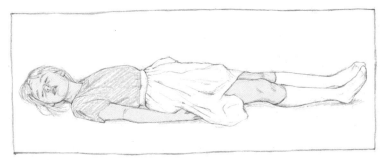

1 Turn your child's head towards you and tilt it back slightly to open the airway. Place the arm nearest you by her side. Lift her bottom and place the hand underneath, palm up with fingers straight.

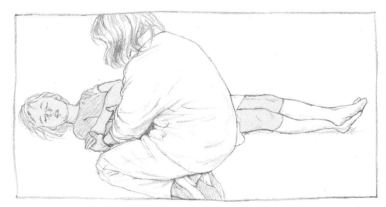

2 Slightly raise the furthest leg at the heel. Then bring it towards you and cross it over the other leg. Bring your child's other arm up and lay it across the front of her chest, in such a way that the hand is pointing towards your child's opposite shoulder.

CHECKING FOR RESPONSE

Your child may pass through various levels of confusion before becoming unconscious and again while regaining consciousness.

Watch her constantly, noting any changes in her state of awareness as this will help the doctor decide on treatment. See if she responds to your voice or to a painful sensation, such as a pinch. If she recovers consciousness, reassure her and get a doctor.

IMPORTANT

▶ If you suspect a fracture, support the fracture but don't put the child into the recovery position.
▶ Continue to check breathing, pulse and level of response every ten minutes.

▶ Never leave your child alone while she is unconscious or give her anything by mouth.
▶ Anyone who has lost consciousness, even for a short time, must be seen by a doctor.

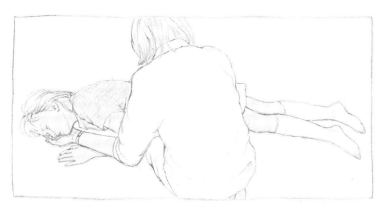

3 Kneel beside your child and support her head with one hand. Grasp her clothes at the hip furthest from you and pull her towards you until she is resting against your knees.

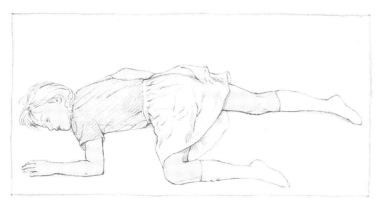

4 Still supporting her body, readjust her head to ensure her airway is open. Bend the uppermost arm and leg to prevent her rolling on to her face. Carefully pull your child's other arm out, working from the shoulder down, and leave it lying parallel to her body.

CONTROLLING SEVERE BLEEDING

Severe bleeding is always an emergency and must be treated as soon as possible. It looks dramatic – blood may be spurting from a wound – but however bad the bleeding looks, don't forget that if your child has stopped breathing, your priority is to open the airway and begin mouth-to-mouth ventilation if necessary (see pages 14–19 for ABC priorities). Then treat the bleeding.

Shock and maybe even death can result from major blood loss. You can help stop the bleeding by pressing directly on the wound and raising the injured part. Watch for signs of internal bleeding (see page 31), such as a large degree of swelling round the injury, sudden, severe pains in the chest or tummy, or the rapid onset of shock.

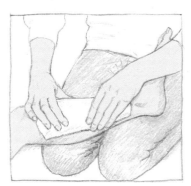

IMPORTANT

▶ Don't remove anything that is embedded in the wound.
▶ Clear away any possible source of further danger, such as shards of broken glass.

1 Apply direct pressure over the wound with your fingers, preferably over a clean pad. Squeeze

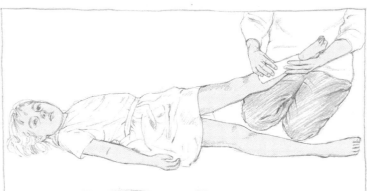

edges of a gaping wound together.

2 Raise and support the injured part above the heart (chest) as you are applying pressure.

3 Place a sterile dressing over the wound so it extends well beyond the wound. Secure firmly with a bandage. Improvise if no dressings are available (see page 54).

4 If blood begins to show through the dressing, don't remove it but put another dressing on top.

5 Watch for shock (see opposite) and get your child to a hospital.

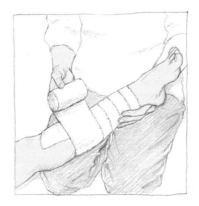

▶ *See page 27 for foreign body in a wound*

▶ *See pages 26–31 for more about bleeding*

DEALING WITH SHOCK

Shock is the result of blood being unable to circulate properly round the body; it is a serious condition which can prove fatal if untreated.

There are many possible causes of shock including electric shock, external or internal bleeding, a severe allergic reaction (anaphylactic shock), or the loss of body fluids after major burns, vomiting or diarrhoea.

If you are not sure whether a child is suffering from shock, or just suspect that it might develop, treat her for shock anyway as a precaution.

Symptoms will become more pronounced as your child's condition deteriorates and include:
● becoming pale and grey, most obviously inside the lips
● skin feels cold and sweaty
● feeling weak and faint
● rapid, weak pulse (normal rate is 80–100 times a minute)
● shallow, fast breathing (normal rate is 20–30 times a minute)
● restlessness, with yawning or sighing
● thirst or vomiting
● unconsciousness

1 Stop any external bleeding by applying direct pressure (see opposite page).

2 Reassure your child and try not to move her. Lay her down, turning her head to one side.

3 Raise her legs, for example by putting folded clothes under her feet. Loosen tight clothing.

4 Keep her warm by wrapping a blanket or coat round her if necessary. Moisten her lips with water, but don't give her a drink.

5 Get an ambulance or medical help as soon as possible.

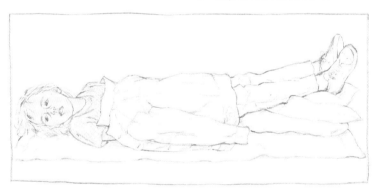

IMPORTANT

▶ Reassure your child and **don't leave her** except to call an ambulance if you are alone.
▶ Don't give her anything to eat or drink, in case she needs to have an anaesthetic.
▶ Never use a hot water bottle to warm your child if she is in shock; it will increase the blood flow to the skin and away from vital organs, such as the heart.

▶ If breathing becomes difficult, place her in the recovery position (see page 20).
▶ If your child becomes unconscious, open her airway and check breathing (see page 14). If necessary, apply mouth-to-mouth ventilation or cardio-pulmonary resuscitation (see pages 16–19). Place her in the recovery position and watch her.

EMERGENCY TREATMENTS

There are many different kinds of emergency you could have to deal with if you have children. In this chapter, you will find information about many of these emergencies: what causes them, what their symptoms are and what treatment you should give.

We refer frequently to the priority techniques described in the previous chapter and you will find that these may be needed in many emergency situations. Keep the ABC priorities in mind at all times:

▶ keep *airway* open
▶ maintain adequate *breathing*
▶ ensure sufficient *circulation*

Remember that you will not necessarily find that the symptoms described as part of each condition will occur in the order given and they may not even all be present in every case.

Try and keep calm and comfort your child if he is conscious. If you have any doubts about his condition, even if he seems fully recovered, take him to a doctor or hospital.

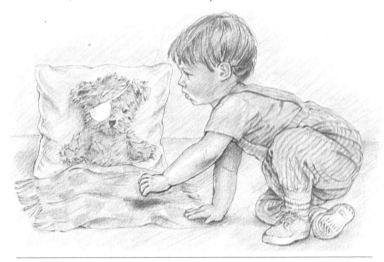

ANAPHYLACTIC SHOCK

This is a massive allergic reaction which can develop very quickly after an insect sting or the injection of a drug to which the child is sensitive. It can also develop as a reaction to a drug such as penicillin.

There are a variety of possible symptoms, amongst them signs of shock (see page 23). Other symptoms include a feeling of nausea, possibly with vomiting; difficulty with breathing; sneezing; swelling of the face, especially round the eyes; rapid pulse; possible unconsciousness.

1 Follow treatment for shock (see page 23) and keep your child's airway open. Place him in the recovery position if his breathing becomes difficult (see page 20).

2 If he becomes unconscious, apply mouth-to-mouth ventilation or CPR if necessary (see pages 16–19). Take him to hospital.

ASPHYXIA

This potentially fatal condition occurs if there is not enough oxygen in the body. Quick treatment is vital; brain cells can die after only three minutes without oxygen. You must restore your child's breathing as quickly as you can.

Causes of asphyxia include:
- food or vomit in the airway
- something heavy compressing the chest
- a fit preventing breathing
- electrical injury
- poisoning
- smoke or gas in the air

Symptoms will include difficulty in breathing; noisy breathing – snoring or gurgling sounds; frothing at the mouth; blueness round the face, lips and fingernails; confusion; lowered level of responsiveness; unconsciousness; breathing may stop altogether.

1 Remove any visible cause of asphyxia and open the airway (see page 14).

2 If your child is conscious and breathing, reassure and watch him, checking breathing and pulse rate (see pages 14–15) and general responsiveness (see page 21) every ten minutes.

3 If your child is unconscious, open his airway and check breathing. Complete the ABC priorities if necessary (see pages 16–19).

4 Get medical help as soon as possible.

SUFFOCATION

This results from an obstruction such as a plastic bag, a pillow or sand preventing air from entering the body. Symptoms are as for asphyxia (see above).

1 Remove the obstruction immediately.

2 If your child is conscious and breathing, reassure him and watch him to make sure his condition does not deteriorate.

3 If he is unconscious, open his airway and check breathing. Complete the ABC priorities if necessary (see pages 16–19).

4 Get medical help as soon as possible.

ASTHMATIC ATTACK

In an asthmatic attack, the small airways of the lungs become narrowed, making a child breathless and wheezy. It particularly affects breathing out. Children who suffer from asthma are usually prescribed a medicine or an inhaler which eases breathing in the event of an attack. Attacks often take place at night, but may occur at any time.

Symptoms of an asthmatic attack are anxiety and difficulty in speaking; breathing difficulty, particularly breathing out; blueness in the face.

1 Reassure and calm the child as he may be frightened.

2 Sit him on a chair or on your lap, leaning slightly forward with his arms supported on something like a table. Make sure there is plenty of fresh air.

3 If he needs medication, either give it to him or if necessary help him to take it.

4 You should take the child to a doctor if the attack continues or keeps recurring.

BLEEDING

Bleeding can occur externally, from an open wound, or internally, when it may be invisible or show as a bruise. External bleeding stops when a clot forms in the wound. You can help this by pressing on to the wound and raising the injured part. However, there are some special types of bleeding where this treatment does not apply (see pages 28–31).

If the wound has been caused by a sharp object such as a needle or a fork (a puncture wound), there is a high risk of the wound becoming infected, so consult your doctor as soon as possible.

However bad the bleeding is, don't forget to check the ABC priorities: ensure an open *airway,* restart *breathing* if necessary and maintain *circulation.* If your child is not breathing or is unconscious, you must treat this before the bleeding or she could die.

IMPORTANT

▶ Major external bleeding can lead to shock (see page 23) and death. You must act quickly to stop the bleeding if a large amount of blood is being lost or if the blood is bright red and spurting regularly. As well as bleeding, your child may show signs of shock.

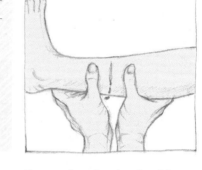

1 Check for foreign bodies (see opposite page). Apply direct pressure by pressing with your thumb or fingers over the wound, ideally over a clean dressing.

Squeeze the edges together if the wound is gaping.

2 Raise and support an injured limb so it is above the heart. If you suspect a fracture, see page 44.

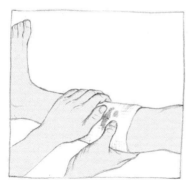

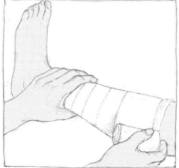

3 Place a sterile dressing over the wound so it extends well beyond the wound's edges. Secure it with a bandage, firmly enough to stop the bleeding but not so tight that it stops circulation. Improvise if you don't have a sterile dressing.

4 If blood starts to show through the dressing, place more dressings on top of the first one and bandage in place.

5 Treat for shock (see page 23) if necessary and get your child to hospital as soon as you can.

▶ *See page 55 for checking circulation*

▶ *See page 59 for minor cuts and grazes*

FOREIGN BODY IN WOUND

Never remove any object, like a piece of glass, embedded in a wound; it may be plugging the wound, so reducing bleeding.

If there are small foreign bodies (for example, pieces of gravel) on the surface of the wound, remove these if they can be easily wiped off or rinsed off with cold water.

1 Control the bleeding by raising the injured part so it is above the heart and by pressing the area that is immediately above and below the wound.

2 Drape a piece of gauze over the wound very gently, taking care not to press down on it.

3 Carefully build up pads of cotton wool or similar material round the foreign body until the pads are at least the same height as the object. Don't pull the gauze down as you do this. If you haven't enough material to build the dressing up to the height of the object, leave it sticking out above the wound.

4 Get a roller bandage and place the end over the part of dressing nearest to you. Make two straight turns, starting on the inside of the limb, then pass the bandage under the limb and bring it up round the other edge of the dressing. Continue alternating turns until the dressing is secure, then fasten the bandage.

5 Keep the injured limb raised and immobilized (see Fractures, page 46).

6 Take your child to hospital as soon as you can.

▶ If your child falls on to spikes or railings and becomes impaled, **do not lift her off.** Support the weight of her limbs and trunk and get someone to call an ambulance immediately. Make sure they explain the nature of the accident to the switchboard operator, so cutting tools can be brought without delay.

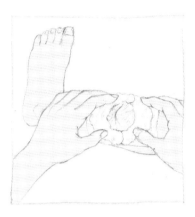

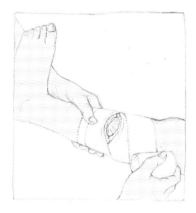

AMPUTATIONS

If your child has an accident which involves the amputation of a limb, finger or toe, there is a chance that doctors will be able to reattach the amputated part if you can get your child to hospital quickly.

1 Control the bleeding by raising the injured part and applying direct pressure (see opposite). Make sure you don't damage the stump when you do this.

2 Place the severed part in a suitable container – a clean plastic bag is ideal. If possible, wrap the bag in some material and put it in a container of ice, making sure the material will prevent the ice from touching against the flesh.

3 Get your child quickly to hospital. When you phone the ambulance service, tell them the nature of the injury so the hospital can be ready to do the appropriate surgery.

SCALP WOUND

Injuries to the scalp – the skin covering the head – are usually the result of falls; other causes include road and sports accidents. Scalp wounds tend to bleed a lot, so the injury will often appear worse than it really is. However, a blow to the head can easily cause concussion or a fractured skull (see Head injuries, page 48), so you must always take your child to a doctor after such an injury.

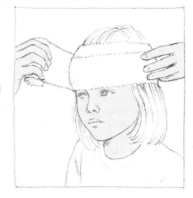

1 Cover the wound with a sterile dressing or clean pad and bandage in place.

2 If your child is conscious, lay her down with her head and shoulders slightly raised and arrange for an ambulance as soon as possible.

3 If your child becomes unconscious, open her airway and check her breathing (see page 14). Complete the ABC priorities if necessary, keeping the injured side up when in the recovery position.

BLEEDING FROM THE EAR

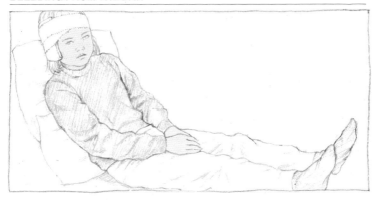

Bleeding from the ear can be the result of either a ruptured eardrum or a fractured skull. Young children often push small objects into their ears and this can rupture the eardrum, causing pain and temporary deafness. If the skull is fractured (see page 48), the blood coming from the ear may be mixed with a clear, straw-coloured fluid. A fractured skull may be the result of a fall or blow to the head and your child may also have a headache and become unconscious.

1 Ease your child into a comfortable position with her head tilted towards the injured side.

2 Cover the whole ear with a sterile dressing and bandage lightly in place, or use adhesive tape to secure it. **Don't** put anything inside the ear to stop bleeding.

3 Watch for signs of shock and treat if necessary (see page 23).

4 If your child becomes unconscious, open her airway and check breathing (see page 14). Complete the ABC priorities if necessary (see pages 16–19), turning her head with the injured side down when in the recovery position.

5 Get her to hospital as quickly as possible.

BLEEDING FROM THE EYE

The eye is very easily damaged and even a superficial graze can scar the surface of your child's eye or lead to an infection.

Your child may suffer loss of vision in the injured eye, or it may be painful and bloodshot; blood or clear fluid may be oozing from it.

If a foreign body is embedded in your child's eye, **don't** attempt to remove it.

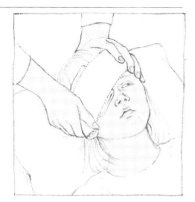

1 Lay your child on her back, supporting her head and keeping it as still as possible.

2 Close the injured eye and gently cover with an eye pad or sterile dressing. Fix it in position with a bandage or some adhesive tape. If your child cannot keep the other eye still, bandage it as well.

3 Get her to hospital as soon as possible.

BLEEDING FROM THE NOSE

Most bleeding from the nose is fairly harmless and the blood comes from the blood vessels inside the nostrils. However, a nosebleed caused by a blow to the face may indicate a fractured nose. Treat the nosebleed (see page 60) and take your child to hospital.

If the bleeding is the result of a blow to the head, or the blood is mixed with a straw-coloured fluid, there is a danger that your child may have fractured her skull (see page 48), so take her to hospital immediately, making sure her airway is kept open.

BLEEDING FROM THE PALM OF THE HAND

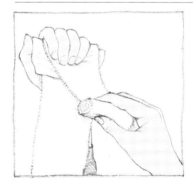

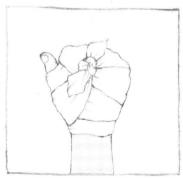

Wounds in the palm tend to bleed a lot and it is sometimes difficult to control the bleeding. **Don't** try and remove any foreign bodies.

1 Raise your child's arm. Place a sterile dressing or gauze and clean pad over the wound and press with your fingers.

2 Get your child to clench her fist tightly over the pad – you may have to help her. Wind the long end of the bandage round the fist, leaving the thumb out for testing circulation. Tie the bandage across the top of the knuckles.

3 Take your child to hospital as soon as possible.

▶ See page 55 for checking circulation

CHEST WOUNDS

A wound which penetrates the chest can be very serious. Air can enter the space normally filled by the lungs, causing the affected lung to collapse and so affect breathing. A wound to the lower chest may cause severe internal bleeding. The wound must be sealed immediately and your child should be taken to hospital as quickly as possible.

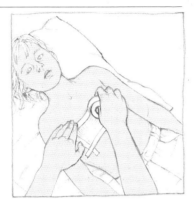

Symptoms may include difficulty in breathing; pain in her chest; signs of asphyxia (see page 25) and shock (see page 23); coughing up bright red frothy blood; sound of air entering her chest as she breathes in.

1 Call an ambulance. Cover the open wound with your palm to seal it and move your child to a half-sitting position, leaning towards her injured side. Comfort her.

2 Cover the wound with a sterile dressing. Use foil or plastic to cover the dressing and make an airtight seal. Keep the dressing in place with adhesive tape or a bandage.

3 Follow the ABC priorities (see pages 14–19) if she becomes unconscious, keeping the injured side uppermost in the recovery position.

ABDOMINAL WOUNDS

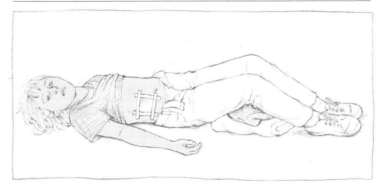

A deep abdominal wound can damage vital organs and cause internal bleeding (see opposite) and possible infection, as well as external bleeding. As well as suffering pain, your child may vomit and show signs of shock (see page 23). Part of the intestine may be sticking out of the wound; if this is the case, do not touch it, but if your child coughs or vomits, press gently on the dressing to prevent the intestines moving. You must protect the wound to reduce the chance of infection, and get your child to hospital.

1 Call an ambulance. Lay your child on her back, with her knees bent up and supported by you.

2 Cover the wound with a sterile dressing or gauze and a clean pad. Keep it in place with a bandage or adhesive tape.

3 Don't give your child anything by mouth.

4 Check for signs of shock (see page 23) and internal bleeding (see opposite page).

5 Follow the ABC priorities (see pages 14–19) if she becomes unconscious.

INTERNAL BLEEDING

Although no blood is lost from the body, internal bleeding results in blood being lost from the circulatory system, starving vital organs of oxygen. It can be caused by a fracture, crush, penetrating injury or hard blow to the body. The blood can collect internally, causing problems if it presses on, for example, the lungs or brain.

There may be no outward sign of internal bleeding. If your child seems to be in shock after a violent injury, although there is no sign of blood, suspect internal bleeding. Pattern bruising, where outlines of clothing are seen in the bruise, may also indicate internal injury. Internal bleeding can lead to some blood being passed from the mouth or anus or in the urine; for example, bright red frothy blood may be coughed up from the lungs.

Other signs of internal bleeding are severe swelling round an injury and sudden severe pains in the chest or tummy.

It is not usually possible to do much to control internal bleeding so you must get your child to hospital as quickly as you can. Don't give her anything by mouth as she will probably need to have an anaesthetic when she reaches the hospital. If possible, keep a sample of any vomit, urine or stool from your child after the injury and take this to the hospital with you.

1 Call an ambulance. Lay your child down with her head low and turned to one side, to encourage the blood supply to the brain. Keep her as still as possible.

2 Check quickly for other injuries and treat as necessary. Depending on what other injuries there are, raise her legs in order to encourage blood to reach the vital organs.

3 Loosen any tight clothing round her neck, chest and waist. Keep

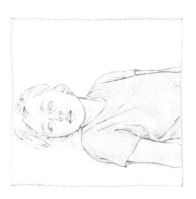

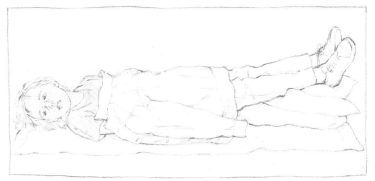

her covered and if possible lay a blanket underneath her.

4 Try and help her relax as much as possible.

5 Stay with your child and check her breathing (see page 14),

pulse (see page 15) and general responsiveness (see page 21) every ten minutes.

6 If your child becomes unconscious, follow the ABC priorities (see pages 14–19).

BURNS AND SCALDS

Burns are a major cause of accidental death among children. They are caused by extremes of temperature (hot and cold), chemicals or radiation. Scalds are burns caused by wet heat such as steam or hot liquids. Electricity is another possible cause of burns (see Electric shock, page 41).

Burns and scalds are serious because, as the skin is broken, they allow infection to enter the body. Superficial burns affect only the surface layers of skin – the skin will become red soon after the burn. Deep burns go though the layers of skin, and the skin may be grey and charred. The other danger is loss of body fluid which can lead to shock. This will develop if more than one tenth of the body surface (an area roughly the size of the stomach) is burned. If more than one third of the body surface is burned, your child's life will be in immediate danger and you must get straight to a hospital. Swelling will also develop around a burn and your child will probably feel severe pain. Consult a doctor if you have any worries about even an apparently minor burn on a baby or young child.

You should contact a doctor or hospital if the burn or scald:

▶ covers an area more than one centimetre (½ in) in diameter
▶ is deeper than the surface of the skin
▶ has been caused by an electrical current
▶ is anywhere on a baby.

Blisters – small bubbles of fluid – may form under the skin after a burn. These are caused by body fluid leaking into the burnt area under the surface of the skin and, during healing, new skin will form under the blister. You should never break a blister on purpose, as this will increase the risk of infection.

IF CLOTHING IS ON FIRE

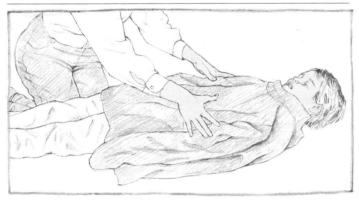

Clothing on fire can lead to major burns, shock and even death. Lay your child down and quickly put out the flames either by using water or another cold liquid such as milk, or by wrapping him tightly in something made from a heavy, non-synthetic fabric, such as a coat, rug or curtain, to smother the flames. Don't roll him over.

GENERAL TREATMENT

When treating a burn or scald, your aim is to cool the area quickly, prevent infection, relieve pain and minimize shock. The treatment of a burn or a scald then depends on the severity of the injury (see page 34 for minor burns).

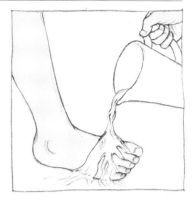

1 Remove your child from any danger, such as an electric fire (see Electricity, page 13), and put out flames if his clothes are on fire (see opposite page).

2 Cool the burnt area. If possible, hold the injured part under cold running water for at least ten minutes to reduce pain. Do this for longer if pain persists. An alternative is to immerse the burnt area in a bucket or bath of cold water, or to pour several jugs of cold water over the burnt area (lay the casualty down before doing this).

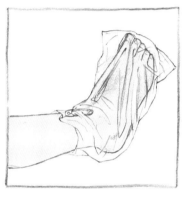

3 Remove any tight clothing, belts or jewellery from the burnt area before it starts to swell. Remove any clothing soaked in boiling liquid after it has begun to cool down. Don't remove anything which is sticking to the burn.

4 Protect the burnt area by covering it with a sterile dressing or clean handkerchief or sheet – anything which is not fluffy will do. If a hand or foot has been burnt, you can cover it with a clean plastic bag. Fix the dressing or bag with a bandage or safety pins; make sure you leave room for any swelling.

5 Immobilize a badly burnt limb (see Fractures, page 46).

6 Treat for shock (see page 23) if necessary.

7 If your child becomes unconscious, follow the ABC priorities (see pages 14–19).

8 Take your child to hospital as soon as you can.

IMPORTANT

▶ Don't break blisters, or remove any loose skin.
▶ Don't remove anything that is sticking to an injury caused by a burn.
▶ Never put fats, lotions or any ointments on a burn.
▶ Don't use adhesive dressings.
▶ Never cover a burn with cotton wool or anything fluffy.
▶ If the burns are on a baby, don't immerse the baby in cold water for too long as this can cause hypothermia.
▶ Don't give your child anything to eat or drink in case an anaesthetic is needed later.
▶ All burns, except very small superficial ones, should be seen by a doctor or in hospital as quickly as possible. Always get medical advice after any burn to a baby or if you are in any doubt at all about the severity of the injury.

TREATMENT FOR MINOR BURNS

You can treat small burns of under one centimetre (½in) across at home (see previous page for when to seek medical help and treatment for more serious burns and scalds).

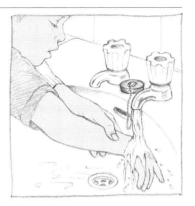

1 Place the burnt area under cold running water or immerse it in cold water in a bath or bucket. Do this for at least ten minutes or until the pain eases. It may take a little while for the tissues under the skin to cool down. Don't immerse a baby for too long.

 If no water is available, you can use any other cold harmless liquid (for example, milk or beer).

2 Gently remove anything like tight clothing, belts or jewellery which may become too tight as the burnt area starts to swell.

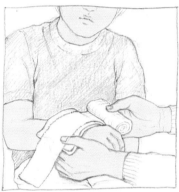

3 Protect the injured area with a sterile dressing large enough to completely cover it (see page 54). If you don't have a dressing, use a handkerchief or anything else that is clean and not fluffy.

4 If you are at all worried, contact a doctor.

SMOKE INHALATION

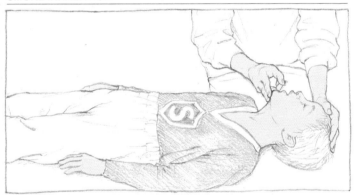

Inhaling smoke can lead to asphyxia (see page 25); you must get your child into fresh air as soon as possible. Don't go into the area where the fire is unless you are sure that there are no toxic fumes (see page 13).

 Put out any clothing that is on fire (see page 32) and, if your child is unconscious, open his airway and check breathing (see page 14). Complete the ABC priorities and treat any burns. Get him to a hospital quickly.

BURNS IN THE MOUTH OR THROAT

Burns in these areas are usually caused by drinking very hot liquid, swallowing corrosive chemicals or inhaling very hot air. The lining of the mouth and throat will swell quickly and may impede the passage of air to the lungs.

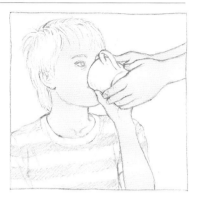

Your child will be in considerable pain and the skin round the mouth may be damaged. He will have difficulty in breathing and may show signs of shock (see page 23) or be unconscious.

Reassure a conscious child and try to stop him from panicking, as this will make it harder for him to breathe.

1 If he is conscious, wash his mouth out with cold water and give him frequent sips of cold water to drink.

2 Remove any tight clothing round the neck and chest.

3 If he becomes unconscious, open the airway and check his breathing and pulse (see pages 14–15). Then complete the ABC priorities (see pages 16–19) if necessary.

4 Get him to hospital as quickly as possible.

CHEMICAL BURNS IN THE EYE

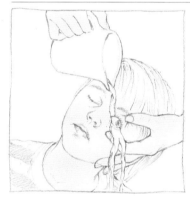

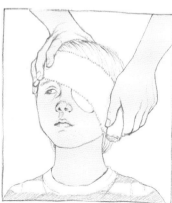

Caustic soda, bleaches, paint stripper or similar materials can seriously damage the skin and eye. You must wash the chemicals off the skin or out of the eye as quickly as possible. Try to avoid coming into contact with the chemical yourself.

If chemicals have gone into your child's eye, he will be in intense pain, and the eye may be tightly closed, reddened, swollen or watering badly. Stop him rubbing the injured eye.

1 Hold the injured side of his face under gently running cold water, so the water drains away from his face, for at least ten minutes. You may find it easier to pour the water from a jug, again making sure that it runs away from the face and the other eye.

If the eye is shut tightly, you may have to gently pull the lid open to wash under it.

2 Dress the eye with an eye pad or a pad of clean, non-fluffy material and bandage it carefully in place.

3 Get your child to hospital as quickly as possible.

CHOKING

Choking occurs when the airway is partially or totally blocked. It can be caused by food going down 'the wrong way', that is, down the windpipe rather than the food passage. With young children and babies, it is often the result of their putting small objects into their mouths and then swallowing the object.

The obstruction must be removed quickly so breathing is restored. Symptoms include blueness of the face; the child will be unable to speak or breathe, and unconsciousness may develop.

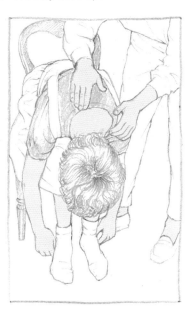

1 Remove anything in your child's mouth with your fingers and get her to cough the obstruction out.

2 If this is unsuccessful, make her bend over so her head is lower than her chest (do this in whatever position you find your child, whether standing or sitting). Slap her firmly between the shoulder blades with the heel of your hand; repeat four times.

3 If the object has not moved, try abdominal thrust (see page 38).

4 Check inside her mouth again. If you can see the obstruction, hook it out with your fingers.

5 If your child is still choking, repeat back slaps and abdominal thrusts, up to four times each.

6 Your child may begin breathing at any stage; when she does, sit her up and give her sips of water.

FOR A YOUNG CHILD

If a young child is choking, the treatment is similar to that for an older child, but using less force.

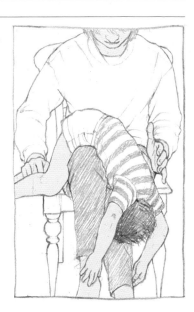

1 Sit in a chair and lay your child across your knees, with his head down.

2 Using one hand to support his chest, slap him firmly between the shoulder blades, up to four times, using your other hand.

3 If this fails to shift the obstruction, you should try using an abdominal thrust (see page 38).

4 If your child becomes unconscious while you are trying to clear his air passages, treat him as described opposite.

5 If your child starts breathing again, sit him up and give him sips of water.

FOR AN UNCONSCIOUS CHOKING CHILD

Choking will lead to unconsciousness if the obstruction is not quickly removed. If this happens, you will have to carry out mouth-to-mouth ventilation to try and get air past the blockage and into your child's lungs.

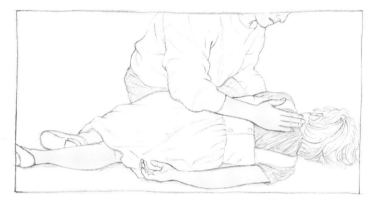

1 Turn the child on her back, open her airway (see page 14) and start mouth-to-mouth ventilation (see page 16).

2 If this doesn't work, turn her on her side, facing you. Supporting her against your thigh, with her head back, do four back slaps.

3 Look to see if the object has been dislodged and hook it out with your finger.

4 If it has not been dislodged, try mouth-to-mouth ventilation again and repeat the above steps. Continue this procedure and send someone to call an ambulance.

5 If you succeed in dislodging the object, place the child in the recovery position while waiting for the ambulance.

FOR A BABY

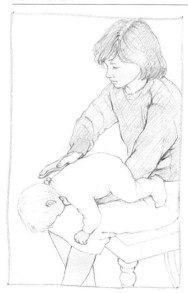

Use only light pressure on a choking baby.

1 Lay the baby along your forearm, face down, so her head is lower than her chest. Use your arm to support her head and chest.

2 Give four light slaps between the shoulders with the other hand. If the object is not dislodged, use abdominal thrust (see page 38).

3 If your baby becomes unconscious, treat as described above, using less force.

4 Sit her up and give her a drink when she starts breathing again.

▶ Only put your finger in your baby's mouth if you can see the obstruction and there is no danger of pushing it further down her throat.

ABDOMINAL THRUST

This technique can be used if back slaps have failed to dislodge an obstruction. However, it can damage internal organs, so use **only** after treatment for choking (see previous page) has failed.

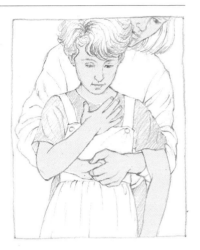

1 Stand behind the child. Clench your fist and place it, thumb inwards, over her stomach between breastbone and tummy button. Grasp your fist with the other hand.

2 Pull both hands towards you with a quick inward and upward movement. Repeat up to four times. The obstruction may shoot into or out of her mouth. Get medical help.

FOR A YOUNG CHILD

Only use abdominal thrust on a young child as a last resort. The thrust must, however, be hard enough to dislodge the obstruction.

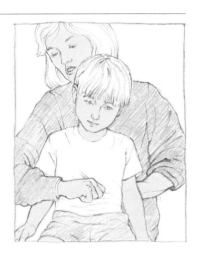

1 Sit your child on your lap or stand him in front of you. Clench your fist and place it, thumb inwards, over his stomach between his tummy button and breastbone. Support his back with your other hand.

2 Press your clenched fist into his stomach with a sudden inward and upward movement. If the thrust fails to dislodge the obstruction, repeat up to four times. Get medical help.

FOR A BABY

As with a young child, you must only use this technique as a last resort for treating choking.

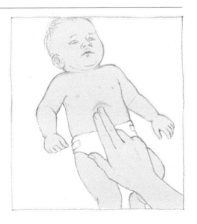

1 Lay your baby on a firm surface with her head in the open airway position (see page 14). Place the first two fingers of one hand on her stomach between her breastbone and tummy button.

2 Press with a quick inward and upward movement, hard enough to dislodge the obstruction. If this fails to dislodge the object, repeat up to four times. Get medical help.

CONVULSIONS

These are fits and are most common in children under five. They can be caused by a very high temperature, a bad tummy upset, a fright or a temper tantrum, or epilepsy.

Convulsions look frightening, but are not dangerous. You must protect your child from hurting herself, though don't try to restrain her.

Symptoms include high fever with a very hot forehead; stiffened body and arched back; twitching muscles; rolling eyes or a squint; her face may look blue if she is holding her breath; froth may appear at her mouth.

1 Loosen any tight clothing and make sure she has plenty of fresh air.

2 Clear a space round her if the convulsions are severe and wipe away any froth.

3 Cool the child by removing any bedding and sponging her down with tepid water. Take care not to let her get too cold.

4 When the convulsions stop, place her in the recovery position and put a light blanket over her. Comfort her and contact your doctor.

DEHYDRATION

Dehydration is the result of an abnormally high loss of salt and water from the body. This can happen as the result of a severe attack of diarrhoea or vomiting or because of heavy sweating.

To avoid dehydration, give children plenty to drink and keep them cool in hot weather. Dehydration can lead to heat exhaustion.

HEAT EXHAUSTION

Symptoms include cramp-like pains and headache; feeling exhausted but restless; dizziness and nausea; pale, moist skin; shallow, fast breathing; rapid, weak pulse.

1 Lay your child down in a cool place. If she is conscious, give her sips of cold water.

2 If she is sweating a lot, has cramps, diarrhoea or vomiting, make sure she keeps drinking as much as possible.

3 If she becomes unconscious, open her airway and check breathing (see page 14). Complete ABC priorities if necessary (see pages 16–19) and get medical help.

DIABETES

With diabetes, a child's body cannot properly regulate the amount of sugar in her blood. Most diabetics carry a card or wear a bracelet.

Comas can be caused by the diabetic child eating too little food or missing a meal; by exercise burning up the sugar; by taking too much insulin. A coma will result in unconsciousness and, if untreated, possibly death.

1 If the child is still conscious and can swallow, give her sugar, chocolate, a sweet drink or similar to raise the level of sugar in her blood. Give more if her condition improves and contact a doctor.

2 If she is unconscious, open the airway and check breathing (see page 14). Complete the ABC priorities if necessary (see pages 16–19) and get medical help as soon as possible.

▶ See page 41 for epilepsy

DROWNING

Drowning causes asphyxia (see page 25) either by water flooding the lungs or by causing the throat to go into spasm, thereby blocking the airway. Quick action can save the victim's life and your priority is to get air into his lungs as fast as possible, if necessary even if you're still in the water. But take care you do not put your life in danger; unless you are a strong and experienced swimmer, you should not attempt a rescue from deep water or where there is a strong current.

Once you have reached the child, start mouth-to-mouth immediately and continue even if you think there is no hope; victims of drowning can take a while to revive. Don't waste time trying to get water out of his lungs. Anyone rescued from drowning should go to hospital.

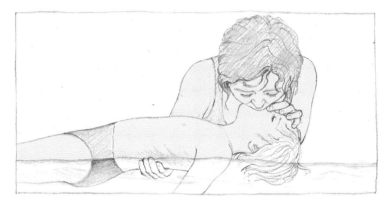

1 Remove any obstructions like seaweed from your child's mouth and begin mouth-to-mouth ventilation (see page 16).

If your child is still in the water, try to start mouth-to-mouth there. In shallow water where you can touch the bottom, support his body with one hand and use the other hand to support his head and seal his nose while you breathe air into his lungs. In deep water, give occasional breaths while getting to shallow water.

2 When you get to dry land, check his breathing and pulse (see page 14); continue mouth-to-mouth ventilation if needed.

3 Place him in the recovery position (see page 20) as soon as he starts breathing. Keep him warm and watch for hypothermia (see page 49).

4 Call an ambulance to take him to hospital.

RESCUING A CHILD

If you are not a good swimmer, there are other ways of rescuing a child. If he is within reach of land, hold a branch or scarf out for him to grasp, making sure you are not pulled in yourself. Try to find someone or something to hold on to while you drag the child in. If you know the water is shallow, wade in to reach the child. In calm, deeper water, a boat could be used; pull the child aboard over the front or back rather than the side to reduce the risk of the boat capsizing. If a child has fallen through ice, test the ice to make sure it will bear your weight. Tell him to stretch his arms forward and kick back in the water to prevent being dragged under. Hold something out for him to hang on to and lie down to pull him in.

ELECTRIC SHOCK

An electric shock may result in severe and sometimes fatal injuries. Babies and young children are particularly at risk because they may play with switches and wiring. Unconsciousness, asphyxia, deep burns and shock can result from an electric shock.

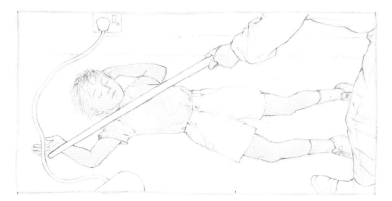

1 Switch off the current at the mains or pull out the plug. If you cannot do this, push the child clear with something insulated such as a wooden chair or broom handle. **Don't** touch the child until the current is broken.

2 If the child is unconscious, open his airway and check breathing (see page 14). Complete the ABC priorities (see pages 16–19) if necessary.

3 Treat any burns (see page 32) and watch for signs of shock (see page 23) if your child is conscious.

4 Get medical help or take your child to hospital.

EPILEPSY

Epilepsy is a tendency to fits or seizures. Minor fits can be almost unnoticed; the child may just seem to be daydreaming. Major fits start with rigidity and loss of consciousness, followed by jerking. Froth may appear round the child's mouth. Fits do not usually last more than five minutes, and the child will naturally regain consciousness, but may be dazed. Don't leave him until he has completely recovered. Seek medical help if he has several fits without regaining consciousness.

1 Lay the child down gently and clear a space round him. Place some soft padding round his head.

2 Carefully loosen any tight clothing round the neck.

3 When the jerking stops, place the child in the recovery position (see page 20).

4 Take the child to your doctor if this is the first attack.

IMPORTANT

▶ Don't try to stop the convulsions or to hold down a child during a fit.
▶ Don't give him anything to eat or drink or put anything in his mouth during the fit.
▶ Don't move him unless he is in danger.
▶ Don't try to wake him.

▶ *See page 13 for electrical hazards*
▶ *See page 32 for burns*
▶ *See page 39 for convulsions*

FOREIGN BODIES

These are small objects that enter the body through a wound or an opening such as the eye, ear or mouth. A foreign body in a wound may sometimes be plugging the wound and preventing blood loss (see page 27). Children often swallow small items, such as coins or beads, or push them up their noses or into their ears. Make sure that your child's tetanus inoculations are kept up to date as there is a high risk of infection from foreign bodies. (See also Splinters, page 61.)

IN THE EYE

Bits of dust or grit, eyelashes or insects are the foreign bodies most commonly found in the eye. They usually stick to the outer surface of the upper eyelid, making the eye painful, watery and red. However, they can be fairly easily removed. **Never** try and remove anything that is on the coloured part of the eye or stuck in the eyeball; if your child has such an injury, cover his eye with a sterile eye pad and take him straight to hospital.

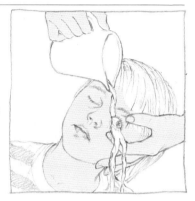

1 Try and stop your child from rubbing his eye.

2 Sit him down in a chair facing the light and lean him back slightly. Wash your hands.

3 Stand behind him, with his head resting against you. Use your thumb and index finger to gently separate the lids and look into his eye. If he is old enough, ask him to look from side to side and up and down so you can see all the eye.

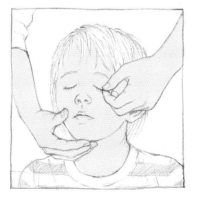

4 If you can see the foreign body, try and wash it out by pouring cold water over the eye. You can use a jug or hold your child's head under the cold tap. Turn his head towards the injured side so the water will drain away from the injured eye.

5 If this doesn't work or there is no water, use a damp swab or corner of a clean handkerchief or tissue to lift the body off.

6 If you think the foreign body is on the upper lid, try and get your child to look down. Holding the lashes of the upper lid, pull the lid down and out over the lower lid.

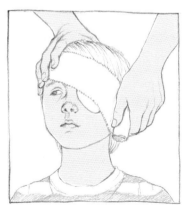

7 If you still haven't succeeded in moving it, cover his eye with an eye pad and take him to the doctor.

▶ See page 27 for foreign body in wound

▶ See page 61 for splinters

IN THE EAR

This is most common in young children, who have a tendency to put small objects into their ears. Your child will have a pain in his ear and his hearing on that side may also be affected. Sometimes an insect may fly into your child's ear and he may then also feel vibrations. Never poke anything inside your child's ear – you could very easily push the insect or object in even deeper, causing damage to the eardrum.

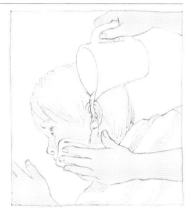

1 Reassure your child as much as you can.

2 If you know it is an insect in his ear, sit your child down or lay him down on his side with the affected ear uppermost. Gently pour tepid water into the ear; the insect should float out.

3 If your child has pushed something into his ear, try tilting his head so that the affected ear is facing downward; the foreign body may then just drop out without any further problem.

4 If you cannot remove the foreign body easily, take your child straight to hospital.

IMPORTANT

▶ Don't try and dig the foreign body out – you could cause further damage.

IN THE NOSE

This is most likely to happen with very young children, who will often try putting things, such as beads, pebbles or marbles, up their noses. If the object is smooth, it may simply become stuck, but a sharp object could damage the delicate tissues in the nose. If something does get lodged, your child may have a swollen nose and difficulty in breathing through his nose; there may also be a discharge.

1 Keep your child as calm as possible and, if he is old enough to understand, tell him to breathe through his mouth. Stop him from rubbing his nose.

2 Don't try and remove the object yourself as you could push it further in. Get your child to a hospital as quickly as you can.

SWALLOWED FOREIGN BODIES

Small children often swallow objects like coins, buttons, pieces of toys (like Lego) or pins. If the object is small and smooth, there is not much cause for concern – it is unlikely to cause choking or damage to the intestines as it passes through your child's body. Sharp objects, however, can cause internal injuries.

Don't let your child run with pens or pencils in his mouth or play with the closures used on plastic bags.

1 If the object has become lodged in your child's throat, he may be choking (see page 36) – treat this as a matter of urgency.

2 Reassure your child if he is upset.

3 Unless you are certain that the swallowed object is unlikely to cause any internal damage, get your child to hospital as quickly as you can. Don't give him anything to eat or drink.

FRACTURES

A fracture is a broken or cracked bone and it is a fairly common injury in childhood. There are two main types of fracture: closed and open. Closed fractures are those where the skin round the injury is not broken; in open fractures, the skin is broken (see opposite page). If you suspect a fracture, do not treat it until you have checked your child's airway, breathing and circulation (see ABC priorities, pages 14–19) and stopped any severe bleeding (see page 22).

Don't move a child with a suspected fracture unless you have to – treat her wherever you find her. If you have to move her, steady and support the injured part first. All fractures should be treated very gently to avoid causing further damage. Phone for an ambulance, except for minor fractures (for example, collar bone) when you could get to hospital by car.

Symptoms and signs may include feeling or hearing the bone snap; intense pain near the injury; tenderness; difficulty in moving the injured part; swelling; deformity, such as a twisted limb; and signs of shock.

GENERAL TREATMENT

1 Call an ambulance and reassure the child.

2 Steady and support the injured part with one hand above and the other below the fracture at the joints.

3 With an open fracture, cover the wound with a piece of sterile gauze or other suitable dressing (see opposite).

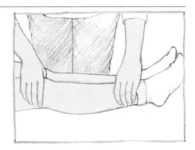

4 If you expect the ambulance to arrive shortly, continue to support the limb and make the child as comfortable as possible.

5 If there is a delay before the ambulance arrives, you should immobilize the broken bone(s). (See pages 46–7 for information on immobilizing specific parts of the body.)

6 Bandage limbs firmly enough to prevent movement, but allow room for some swelling. Check circulation of the bandaged part (see page 55).

7 Raise the affected limb, if possible, to reduce bleeding and swelling. Watch for signs of shock (see page 23) and treat if necessary.

TRACTION

If a limb is bent or broken so awkwardly that it cannot easily be moved for splinting, apply traction to bring it into line. This means exerting a continuous pull on the supported limb as you straighten it. Pull in a straight line, away from the body until the limb is immobilized. Only apply gentle traction and stop if there is *any* resistance.

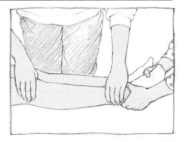

▶ *See page 48 for skull fracture*

OPEN FRACTURES

With an open fracture, the skin is broken and the bone will either stick out through the skin or a wound will open on to the fractured bone. There will almost certainly be bleeding, but the greatest danger is that germs can enter the bone, causing infection, so always get medical help as soon as possible. Open fractures can be caused either by fragments of bone breaking out through the skin or by external force, for example if the child has been hit by a car or flying object.

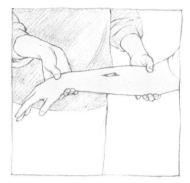

Ideally, two people are needed to treat an open fracture: one to support the injured limb and the other to apply the dressing. The person supporting the injured limb should hold it at the joints above and below the fracture site. Get medical help as soon as possible.

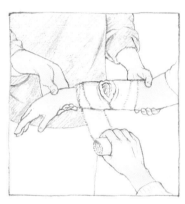

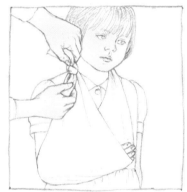

If the bone is protruding:

1 Drape sterile gauze over the exposed bone and pad *round* it with cotton wool. Build up the padding and bandage as in steps 3 and 4 for dressing a wound with a foreign body (see page 27).

2 Immobilize and raise the limb if possible (see pages 46–7).

If the bone is not protruding:

1 Place sterile gauze or other suitable dressing over the wound.

2 Put pads of cotton wool over and round the wound and secure with a roller bandage.

3 Immobilize and raise the limb if possible (see pages 46–7).

IMPORTANT

▶ Any kind of fracture may be complicated by injury to blood vessels, nerves or internal organs, caused by fractured bone ends or fragments.

▶ If you have any doubts about the severity of your child's injury, for example you are uncertain if it is a dislocation or fracture, always treat it as a fracture.

ARM FRACTURE

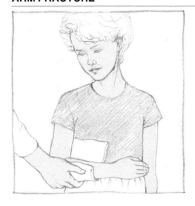
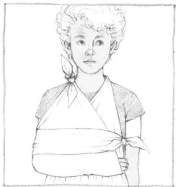

1 Gently bend your child's arm at the elbow and place padding between her arm and body. Support the arm with a sling (see page 57).

▶ If the arm will not bend, lay your child down and place soft padding between her arm and body. Bandage

2 Tie a broad-fold bandage (see page 56) round her trunk to immobilize her arm, avoiding bandaging over the break.

her arm to her body with three broad-fold bandages, avoiding bandaging over the break.

LEG FRACTURE

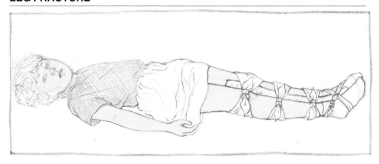

For a fracture below the knee:

1 Steady and support the injured limb by holding at the knee and ankle joints.

2 Immobilize the injured leg by splinting it to the sound one, making sure you move the sound limb towards the injured one and not vice versa.

3 Place three broadly folded triangular bandages under the legs at the knees and above and below the fracture. Put a narrowly folded bandage under the ankles.

4 Fill hollows and cushion ankles and knees with padding. Knot the broad-fold bandages over the uninjured leg and tie the ankle

bandage in a figure-of-eight. Watch for signs of shock (see page 23) and treat if necessary.

For a fracture above the knee:

1 Steady and support by holding at knee and hip joints.

2 If the ambulance is delayed, gently straighten the lower leg and bring the injured leg into line, using traction if necessary (see page 44).

3 Bandage at ankles, knees and above and below fracture, as in steps 3 and 4, left.

▶ Never leave a broken leg unsupported.

RIB FRACTURES

Broken ribs are naturally splinted by being attached to the rest of the rib cage. As well as the usual symptoms of a fracture, your child may have a very sharp pain in her side, made worse by coughing or taking deep breaths, and feel particularly tender around the affected ribs.

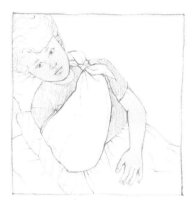

1 Sit your child down and support the arm on the injured side with an arm sling (see page 57).

2 Take her to hospital as soon as possible.

If the fracture is complicated:

The injury may be more serious, involving damage to several ribs and/or the chest wall (see if there is a chest wound or if part of the chest has lost its rigidity). There may be breathing difficulties and possible asphyxia.

1 Treat any serious chest wound first (see page 30).

2 Help your child into a half-sitting position, leaning towards her injured side.

3 Support her arm on the injured side with an elevation sling (see page 57) and wait for the ambulance.

COLLAR BONE FRACTURES

These are most commonly caused by falling on to an outstretched hand or the point of the shoulder. Symptoms and signs may include a reluctance to move the arm on the injured side and a swelling or deformity. Your child will probably be supporting her arm on the injured side and may also be inclining her head towards that side.

1 Place the arm on your child's injured side across her chest, fingertips almost resting on the opposite shoulder.

2 Support the arm in an elevation sling (see page 57) and place soft padding between her upper arm and chest.

3 Secure your child's arm to her chest by tying a broad-fold bandage (see page 56) across the sling and round her body. Tie in front on the uninjured side.

4 Take your child to hospital as soon as possible.

SPINAL INJURIES

A fractured spine can be caused by a child falling awkwardly and landing on her back. Your child may feel tender round the injured part; feel shooting pains in his limbs and/or trunk; be unable to feel or move her legs if the injury is to the lower back and unable to move any limbs if the injury is near the neck.

A fractured spine is a very serious injury. It can be made much worse by incorrect handling and serious disability can result, so if you suspect a child's neck or spine is fractured, **don't move her** unless her life is in danger.

1 Make the child comfortable in the position in which you found her and tell her to keep as still as possible.

2 Hold her head still with your hands and put blankets or pillows along her body and legs; cover her with a blanket.

3 Loosen any tight clothing and wait for the ambulance. Comfort and reassure the child.

HEAD INJURY

Children frequently have falls which result in a bang on the head and in most cases there is no major injury. But there are several serious conditions which can result from a blow to the head, so always watch your child closely after a head injury and consult your doctor.

Any blow to the head which is hard enough to cause a bruise or bleeding could also fracture the skull. Concussion – a temporary shake up of the brain – is another danger; this can also be caused by indirect force, such as a blow to the jaw. Compression – where pressure is exerted on the brain by blood accumulating within the skull or by pressure from a fractured skull – is a very serious condition and can follow concussion; it may develop some hours or days after the child has apparently recovered.

CONCUSSION

This is accompanied by a brief or partial loss of consciousness; on recovery your child may feel sick or vomit. If he is unconscious, treat as on page 20. Check his breathing and pulse rates (see pages 14–15). Watch for signs of compression (see below) and take him to the doctor.

COMPRESSION

If compression is developing, your child's level of responsiveness will deteriorate; his breathing becomes noisy; his pupils may be of different sizes; one side of his body may be weak or paralysed. To test responsiveness, pinch the back of his hand to see if he feels pain. Arrange for your child to get to hospital urgently; treat for unconsciousness (see page 20) and shock (see page 23). Keep his airway well open.

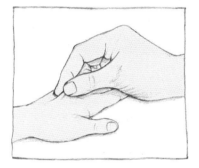

SKULL FRACTURE

Symptoms of a fractured skull include blood or straw-coloured, blood-stained fluid from the ear or nose; bruising on eyelids or white of eye; bleeding from scalp; soft boggy area or depression of scalp; pupils may be of different sizes; very slow pulse.

If any of these symptoms are present, get your child to a hospital quickly, making sure his airway is kept open.

Place him in the recovery position. If an ear is bleeding, cover it with a soft pad; bandage lightly and turn his head so that side is down.

Treat for unconsciousness (see page 20) and apply ABC priorities if

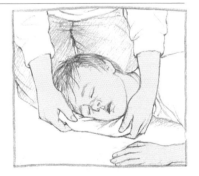

required. Check breathing and pulse rate (see pages 14–15) and level of responsiveness (see above). Watch for signs of compression (see above).

▶ See page 20 for unconsciousness

HEATSTROKE

This happens when the body is unable to control its temperature by sweating, and can occur in hot, humid weather when there is no wind.

Symptoms include restlessness; headache and dizziness; flushed, hot, dry skin; fast, strong pulse; and a temperature of 40°C (104°F) or more. The child may also lose consciousness rapidly.

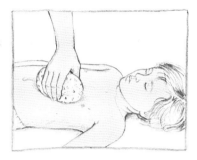

1 Lay your child down in the coolest place possible and take off his clothes.

2 Sponge him down with cold or tepid water.

3 Fan his body by hand or with an electric fan. Continue to fan and sponge him until his temperature falls to 38°C (101°F).

4 Cover him with a dry sheet and get medical help urgently.

HYPOTHERMIA

Hypothermia results when the body temperature drops below 35°C (95°F). Small babies are particularly at risk from hypothermia if a house is badly heated; it can also be caused by lengthy immersion in cold water or by not being dressed warmly enough in cold weather.

As well as low temperature, other symptoms include: cold, pale, dry skin; shivering; clumsy movements and slurred speech; gradual unconsciousness.

A baby with hypothermia will look healthy, but will be unusually quiet and limp, and refuse food.

It is best to rewarm someone with hypothermia at the speed at which they cooled down, that is you should quickly rewarm a child rescued after falling in the sea and gradually rewarm a baby who has become chilled overnight.

1 Replace any wet clothing with dry and put the child in a previously warmed bed.

2 Place a covered hot water bottle in his left armpit or over his breastbone. Do not put hot water bottles on other parts of his body.

3 To rewarm him faster, place in a hot bath of approximately 43 °C (110°F) – the water should be bearable when tested with your elbow.

4 Give him hot drinks and high energy food like chocolate.

5 Get medical attention urgently, particularly for a baby.

If outside

1 Shelter the child as much as possible; put him on a rug and wrap a rug or coat around him. Lie beside him or cuddle him on your lap so your body heat warms him.

2 Get him to hospital as soon as possible.

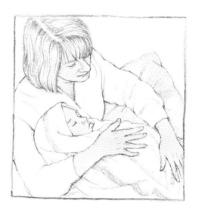

POISONING

A poison is any substance which can produce temporary or permanent damage to the body if taken in sufficient quantity. A poison can be swallowed, breathed in, injected or absorbed through the skin.

There are lots of things in most homes that are poisonous; bleach, white spirit, cleaning materials, glue, shoe polish, insecticides, liquid soap and medicines are just some of them. Children are at particular risk from such materials as they will be unaware of the effects of eating or drinking them. Keep all medicines, cleaning materials and insecticides out of children's reach and in clearly marked containers.

Symptoms will vary depending on the particular poison. Signs to look for are: a container near the child, known to hold or have held a poison; vomiting or diarrhoea; fits; burns on the lips; asphyxia; unconsciousness.

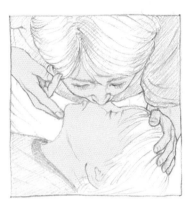

1 Call a doctor or ambulance immediately and tell them what has happened. You must try and keep your child's airway open and maintain his breathing and circulation (see page 14).

2 If your child is conscious, ask him what happened; if he becomes unconscious, follow the ABC priorities (see pages 14–19).

3 Place him in the recovery position (see page 20) even if he is conscious in case he vomits. **Don't** try to make him sick.

4 If mouth-to-mouth ventilation is necessary, wash any poison from your child's face first, to avoid getting any on yourself, or, closing the child's mouth, use mouth-to-nose ventilation (see pages 16–17).

CORROSIVE POISONING

Corrosive poisons may burn the lips, mouth and stomach, causing severe stomach pain. The lips may show signs of burning and be blistered.

If you suspect corrosive poisoning, never try and make your child sick – the poison will burn him again as it is vomited up. When the lips or mouth show signs of burning, cool them by giving your child sips of milk or water to drink.

Make sure you don't come into contact with the poison yourself; either wash it off your child's face before giving mouth-to-mouth ventilation or give mouth-to-nose ventilation, keeping the child's mouth closed (see pages 16–17).

IMPORTANT

▶ Make sure all containers with poisonous substances in them are clearly marked and kept locked up, out of children's reach.
▶ Take care not to get any of the poison on yourself.

▶ Never try and make your child sick after poisoning.
▶ Don't leave your child alone.
▶ When he goes to hospital, take any tablets, medicines or containers found near him.

DRUG POISONING

To reduce the risk of drug poisoning, lock medicines and tablets away. Some of the most dangerous medicines include tablets which look very similar to sweets; these include tranquillizers and other depressants, and some iron tablets. An aspirin overdose is also very dangerous, as is 'glue-sniffing'. Symptoms will vary; your child may vomit and his pupils may be very dilated or contracted.

Depressants will produce shallow breathing; cold, clammy skin; weak and rapid pulse; possible unconsciousness.

Stimulants, such as amphetamines, will make your child excitable with possible tremors and hallucinations; he will be sweating a great deal.
Aspirin overdose produces stomach pain, possibly with vomiting; drowsiness; 'ringing' in the ears; breathing difficulties; sweating.

▶ If you suspect that your child has taken some tablets or medicine, follow the general treatment for poisoning (see opposite page) and get your child to hospital quickly. Be ready to resuscitate him if he should become unconscious.

CARBON MONOXIDE POISONING

Carbon monoxide is a colourless, odourless gas which is easily absorbed by the blood, thus replacing oxygen and causing asphyxia. Car exhaust fumes are the most common source of carbon monoxide, but it can also occur in household heating appliances and when other fuels such as paraffin or gas are burnt.

   Never leave your car engine running in an enclosed space. If your car exhaust system is defective, carbon monoxide will be produced. Take care if you are attempting to rescue your child from, for example, a fume-filled garage (see Hazardous situations, page 13).

Symptoms of carbon monoxide poisoning include signs of asphyxia; headache; skin colour changing to cherry pink as the amount of carbon monoxide in the blood rises; confusion and lack of co-operation; breathing difficulties; unconsciousness. You must restore fresh air and breathing, and then get your child to hospital.

1 Quickly drag your child into the fresh air.

2 Open doors and windows to disperse fumes; switch off car engine or heating appliance.

3 If your child is unconscious, open his airway and check his breathing (see page 14); complete the ABC priorities if necessary (see pages 16–19). You may need to continue mouth-to-mouth ventilation for some time.

4 Get your child to hospital as quickly as possible.

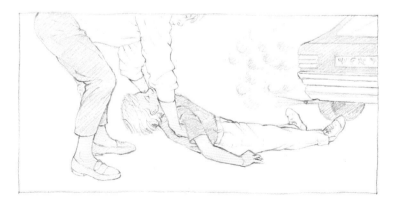

FIRST AID EQUIPMENT

It's a good idea to keep all your first aid equipment together; store items in a clean airtight container, such as a tin or a plastic or wooden box. Label it clearly and keep it in a dry place – in the bathroom is not a good idea, as it will get too steamy. Put the box somewhere easily accessible to adults, but out of reach of children, and don't lock it (you may not be able to find the key in an emergency). Remember to tell anyone looking after your child where the equipment is kept.

You can buy everything you need for a first aid box from most high street chemists or you can choose a pre-packed kit. When you have used something from the box, make sure you replace it. Check all the items every six months or so to make sure they are in good condition.

What you need

1. Small packs of white paper tissues.
2. Scissors, with blunt ends.
3. Tweezers, with blunt ends.
4. Selection of safety pins, including large ones.
5. Clinical thermometer or feverscan forehead thermometer. A clinical thermometer is more accurate, but a forehead thermometer can be quicker and easier to use on a young child.
6. Adhesive dressing (plasters) in various shapes and sizes, some waterproof.
7. Pre-packed sterile dressings (with roller bandage attached), in a variety of different sizes for use on open wounds.
8. Pre-packed burns dressings.
9. Pre-packed sterile gauze, for use on open wounds, for covering foreign bodies or protruding bones, and as an alternative to cotton wool for cleaning cuts and grazes.
10. Roll of cotton wool. This can be used with soap and water for cleaning cuts and grazes; for making a cold compress for a sprain; for using on top of a dressing to soak up blood; for cushioning an injured arm when putting it in a sling; for protecting bones and joints when splinting an arm to the body or an

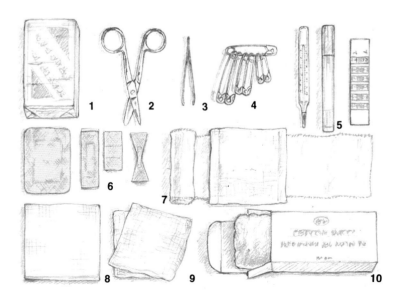

On the inside of the lid, tape a piece of paper with the name, address and phone number of your doctor and the nearest hospital casualty department. Add the same details about friends or neighbours who could be contacted for help in an emergency.

The list below shows what you should try and keep in your home first aid kit. Remember you can improvise bandages and slings from whatever you have to hand, for example, large handkerchiefs or tea towels, but make sure that you have a supply of sterile dressings.

Don't forget to keep some first aid equipment in the car and to take some on holiday with you. A basic kit for the car should include several different-sized sterile dressings; a variety of sticking plasters; a triangular bandage; cotton wool; a packet of antiseptic wipes; a couple of crepe bandages; a selection of different-sized safety pins; tweezers and scissors.

This car first aid kit is also suitable for taking on holiday. Don't forget to add one or two appropriate extras, such as sun screen, calamine lotion and insect repellent.

injured leg to the other leg.

11. Rolled gauze bandage, to keep dressings in place.

12. Adhesive tape, to keep dressings in place or to secure bandages.

13. Rolled crepe bandages, for sprains.

14. Sterile eye pad.

15. Several large linen or cotton triangular bandages, for making a sling or folded bandage to immobilize an injured arm against the body or an injured leg against the other leg. Store these already folded so you can use them straight away in an emergency.

16. Calamine lotion, for soothing bites, stings or sunburn when the skin is not broken and weeping.

17. Witch hazel, for soothing cuts, grazes, bruises, sprains, sunburn and insect bites.

18. Antiseptic lotion or antiseptic wipes, as an alternative to soap and water for cleaning dirty cuts and grazes.

19. Antiseptic cream, for splinters or infected wounds.

20. Junior paracetamol, in liquid or tablet form, depending on the age of your child. Don't give paracetamol to babies under three months.

21. Antihistamine cream, to reduce swelling caused by stings.

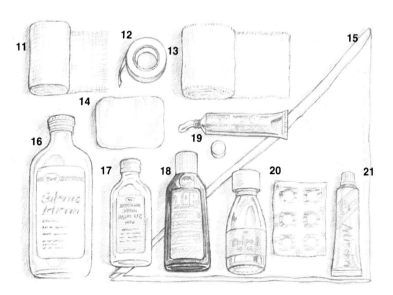

DRESSINGS AND BANDAGES

There are lots of different kinds of dressings and bandages; the type used and the way you use it varies according to the particular injury you are dealing with.

Dressings and bandages are sold in sterile packs. If you don't have any, you can improvise with a clean handkerchief, tea towel or similar non-fluffy material. Don't let whatever you use touch anything before you put it on the wound. Never put fluffy material on an open wound because the fibres will stick to the wound.

Always wash your hands before dressing an open wound. If the bleeding is under control, clean the wound and the surrounding skin; avoid touching the wound or any part of the dressing which will be in contact with the wound. Put the dressing directly on to the wound and if it slips off before you have secured it, use a fresh dressing. Don't talk or cough over the wound or dressing.

Adhesive dressings (plasters) are best for small cuts and grazes. They consist of a small pad attached to an adhesive backing. Make sure the skin around the cut is dry or the plaster will not stick.

STERILE DRESSINGS

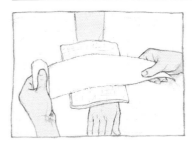 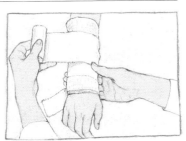

These are the best things to use for large wounds. The dressing consists of layers of gauze or lint and a pad of cotton wool attached to a roller bandage. They come in a variety of shapes and sizes.

Hold the edge of the folded dressing and roller bandage in one hand and unwind the short bandage. Place it gauze side down on the wound. Wind the short bandage once round the limb and dressing then, leaving that end hanging, bandage firmly with the rolled end. Tie ends securely over the pad with a reef knot.

COLD COMPRESS

You must cool injuries like bruises and sprains to minimize swelling and reduce pain. If you cannot easily cool the injury under cold running water, apply a cold compress for about 30 minutes.

1 Soak a pad of cotton wool or towelling in cold or iced water, squeeze it out and place on the injury.

2 Replace or refresh the compress every ten minutes.

3 If it helps, lightly bandage the compress to keep it in position.

▶ An alternative is to use an ice bag. Fill a plastic bag half full of ice and add a little salt (to make the ice melt faster). Squeeze the air out of the bag and seal it. Wrap the bag in a thin towel and hold it over the injury.

BANDAGING

The two main types of bandage are roller bandages and triangular bandages. Roller bandages are used to keep dressings in place, apply pressure to control bleeding, or for a strain or sprain. A triangular bandage is used for slings and, when folded, for immobilizing a fractured limb or for securing dressings in place.

Bandaging is easier than it sounds. It is a good idea to practise bandaging techniques on a healthy limb before you have to do it in a real emergency. You should always stand in front of the injured person when putting on a bandage and support the limb or part of the body in the position in which it is to stay. The bandage needs to be firm enough to hold the dressing in place or control bleeding, but not so tight that it stops circulation (see below). Once you have finished bandaging, check frequently to make sure that it isn't becoming too tight as the injured area swells.

CHECKING CIRCULATION

You should do this as soon as you have put on the bandage and then every ten minutes or so.

To check circulation, press one of the nails or skin of the bandaged limb until it turns white. When you release the pressure the area should quickly become pink again as the blood returns.

If the nail remains white or blue or the fingers are unnaturally cold, the bandage is too tight.

REEF KNOTS

When tying the ends of a bandage, always use a reef knot; it won't slip, lies flat and is easy to untie. If you are using it on a sling, make sure that the knot doesn't press on a bone or into the skin.

1 Hold one end of the bandage in each hand. Take the left end over the right and under.

2 Take the right end over the left and under. Pull the knot firm.

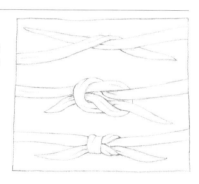

ROLLER BANDAGE

Before you start, make sure the bandage is tightly rolled. Stand in front of your child and support the area to be bandaged in the position in which it is to remain.

The most common method of applying a roller bandage is to use spiral turns. Make a firm straight turn to start, holding the rolled part uppermost. Working up the limb from below the injury, make a series of spiral turns, each one covering two-thirds of the previous one. Finish with a straight turn and secure the end

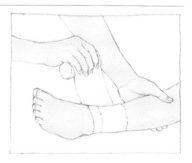

with a safety pin, adhesive tape or bandage clip.

BANDAGING A WRIST (adapt this for an ankle)

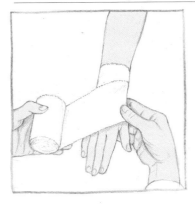 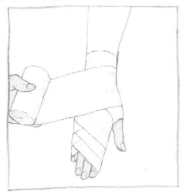

Fix the bandage with one straight turn round your child's wrist. Take the bandage diagonally across the back of her hand towards the base of the little finger, round the palm and under the fingers.

Carry the head of the bandage across the top of the fingers to the nail of the little finger; then bring it down round the palm again and diagonally across the back of the hand towards the wrist. Continue until the hand is covered. Finish with a spiral turn and secure the end.

BANDAGING A KNEE (adapt this for an elbow)

Support your child's knee in a comfortable position – get her to do this herself if she is old enough. Put the tail of the bandage on the inside of her knee and make one straight turn, carrying the bandage head over the knee cap and then right round the leg.

Take the bandage round the thigh, covering half the first turn, then round the calf, covering the outer edge of the first turn and touching the edge of the second turn. Continue turns above and below the knee, with each turn covering just a little more than two-thirds of the previous one. Finish with one or two spiral turns above the

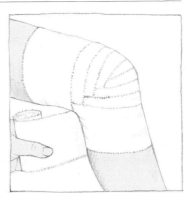

knee and then secure the end of the bandage.

TRIANGULAR BANDAGES

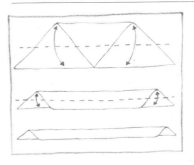

Broad-fold bandage
To make a broad-fold triangular bandage, fold the point down to the base of the bandage and fold in half again.

Narrow-fold bandage
If you fold this bandage again, to make a narrow-fold bandage, you can use it instead of a roller bandage to secure a dressing round an ankle or other joint.

SLINGS

There are two types of slings, arm and elevation. For a small child, fold the triangular bandage in half so the sling is not too big.

ARM SLING

These are for injuries to the upper arm or to immobilize the arm if there is a severe chest injury; they are only effective if your child can sit or stand. You must keep the arm supported until the sling is secure.

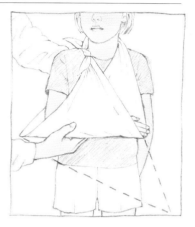

1 Support your child's arm, with wrist slightly higher than elbow.

2 Slide one end of the triangular bandage between arm and chest, with the point well beyond the elbow.

3 Pull the upper end round the back of the neck. Bring the other end up over the forearm. Check that the child's hand is still higher than her elbow and that just her fingertips are exposed. Secure the bandage near the collar bone on the injured side with a reef knot.

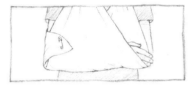

4 Pin the point to the front of the bandage with a safety pin.

ELEVATION SLING

This is used if the hand is bleeding, if there are complicated chest injuries, or if there are shoulder injuries.

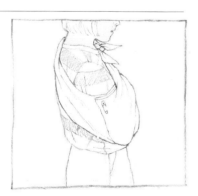

1 Place your child's forearm across her chest, with her fingertips almost resting on her opposite shoulder. Ask her to support it if she can.

2 Place a triangular bandage over her forearm and hand, with the point well beyond the elbow and the upper end just over the shoulder on the uninjured side.

3 Supporting the injured arm, ease the bottom of the bandage under her hand, forearm and elbow.

4 Take the lower end across her back to the front of the uninjured shoulder and tie with a reef knot in front of the hollow above her collar bone.

5 Tuck the point between the forearm and front part of the bandage and secure with a safety pin.

▶ There are ways of improvising slings if you don't have a triangular bandage. You could use a scarf or belt, pin the sleeve of the injured arm to clothing, support it in a jacket opening or turn up the lower edge of a jacket and pin it.

FIRST AID FOR COMMON INJURIES

Animal bites
An animal bite can leave a deep wound and germs can be injected under the skin. If the skin is broken, you must clean it immediately to prevent infection. For a superficial bite, wash the wound with soap and water or a mild antiseptic for five minutes, then dry it and cover with a sterile dressing before contacting your doctor.

If the wound is more serious, you must first control any severe bleeding (see page 22), then cover the wound with a sterile dressing and bandage securely before taking your child to hospital.

There is a risk of tetanus from animal bites, so check your child's immunization record to make sure it is up to date – ask your doctor if you are unsure. To reduce the risk of dog bites, teach your child not to pat or stroke a strange dog, however friendly the dog seems. Tell older children not to run away if a dog starts to chase them, but to try and stay calm and call for help or walk slowly away. Report all dog bites to the police and isolate the animal if you can do so without putting yourself at risk.

If your child – or any adult – is bitten by a dog, cat or monkey when you are abroad, there is a risk of rabies. Rabies is potentially fatal and you must contact a doctor straight away.

Bites and stings see Animal bites, Insect bites and stings, Jellyfish stings, Snake bites

Black eye see Bruising

Bleeding lip or tongue
Bleeding from the lip, tongue or lining of the mouth can start after a fall or blow to the face. The bleeding is usually caused by the teeth.

There is often a lot of blood from this type of cut. This may frighten your child so give him plenty of comfort and stop him swallowing the blood. If the bleeding is not severe, wipe the blood away with tissues. With severe bleeding, place a clean dressing over the cut and squeeze it between your thumb and finger. Do this for ten minutes if you can, allowing him to dribble out any blood in the mouth while you hold the cut.

If the cut is still bleeding badly after ten to twenty minutes, carefully remove the dressing, disturbing the blood clot as little as possible, and use a fresh dressing to continue the pressure for another ten minutes. Take your child to the doctor if the wound is still bleeding after this.

Bleeding tooth socket
This can happen after your child has had a tooth accidentally knocked out or after one of his first teeth has fallen out naturally. Turn his head towards the side that is bleeding and put a thick pad of gauze or clean cloth across – but not in – the tooth socket. Either get your child to bite hard on the pad for ten to twenty minutes or hold the pad in place yourself. If bleeding persists, take him to the dentist. If a tooth has been knocked out, take your child to the dentist as soon as possible. If you can find the tooth, take it with you in a container of milk.

Blisters
Blisters develop after the skin has been damaged by rubbing or a burn. The blister will go down by itself and the skin become dry and fairly hard, eventually falling off.

If the blister is somewhere where it will be rubbed, such as the heel, cover it for a few days with a small gauze pad kept in place with adhesive tape.

If a blister caused by rubbing is still giving your child a lot of discomfort after you have covered it, you could break it. First wash the blister with soap and water. Then sterilize a needle by passing it through a small flame; don't wipe the soot away or touch the end of the needle. When the needle has cooled, pass it through the blister making two holes. Place some clean cotton wool on the blister and press out the fluid. Don't remove the skin, but cover the blister with a plaster. **Never** break blisters caused by a burn.

Pain or inflammation around the blister may mean it is infected, so take your child to the doctor.

Breath-holding

Breath-holding attacks can be frightening for an adult to watch, but they only continue for a limited time. Your child will take a breath as soon as he becomes short of oxygen, although his face might be quite blue before then.

If you want to stop the attack, try blowing gently on to his face or pinching his nostrils together for a second or two.

Bruising

A bruise is bleeding under the skin caused by a sprain or a knock. The area round the bruise often swells up. Most children bruise themselves often and it is usually not serious.

You can minimize the swelling and pain by applying a cold compress (see page 54) and by raising the injured part – on a cushion or in a sling, for example.

A bruise may indicate a broken bone or internal injury, so if you are in any doubt about the severity of the injury or if your child continues to feel severe pain in the area round the bruise, consult your doctor.

A black eye is a bruise caused by a blow to the face. As the eye is so delicate, any blow hard enough to cause a black eye may also lead to eye damage or even a fractured skull. Relieve the pain with a cold compress (see page 54) and take your child to your doctor as soon as you can.

Burns and scalds

Minor burns and scalds can be treated at home, but most burns and scalds will require medical attention – see pages 32–5 for treating burns and scalds.

Cramp

Cramp is a sudden, painful contraction of a muscle or group of muscles. Cramp may be caused by your child getting cold after or during exercise such as swimming or by the loss of salt or fluids from his body through severe sweating, diarrhoea or persistent vomiting. If your child gets cramp, you must try and relax the contracted muscles to relieve the pain. Straighten the affected part of his body and gently massage it. Your child will probably be tense from pain and fright, making the cramp worse, so reassure him that it is not serious.

Crushed finger

Fingers trapped in doors or drawers are a common but painful injury to children. Comfort your child and give him plenty of time to get over the fright and pain. In many cases the pain and swelling can be helped by putting his hand under cold running water or applying a cold compress (see page 54). If the nail is injured or torn, cover the finger loosely with a clean handkerchief and take your child to the doctor.

Cuts and grazes

You can treat small cuts and grazes yourself at home, but larger injuries and severe bleeding (see pages 26–31) will need proper medical treatment.

To minimize the risk of infection, you must first clean the cut or graze and then dress it. You will need cotton wool, soap and water.

First, wash your hands. If the wound is dirty, rinse it under cold running water and clean round it with soap and water, wiping away from the wound. Use a fresh piece of cotton wool for each stroke and try not to disturb any blood clots. Carefully remove any loose dirt.

Dry the area round the wound and cover it with an adhesive dressing.

If the wound starts to ooze or becomes sore and inflamed, consult your doctor.

Dislocation

A dislocation is the displacement of a bone at a joint – most commonly the shoulder, thumb, finger or jaw. It's often difficult to tell if an injury is a dislocation or fracture and if you are in any doubt, treat it as a fracture (see pages 44–7). If your child has dislocated a joint, he will be in severe pain and won't be able to move that part of his body. There may be some swelling round the joint and it may look deformed.

Never try and replace a bone in its normal position as you may only cause further damage. Help your child into a comfortable position, supporting the injury with pillows, blankets or a sling as appropriate. Then call an ambulance. Comfort your child and keep him still.

Fainting

Small children rarely faint. If they do, it's usually due to a nasty fright.

Lay your child down with his head low and feet raised. Loosen any tight clothing round his neck, chest or waist and make sure he's getting plenty of fresh air.

Comfort and reassure him as he regains consciousness. Don't give him anything to drink until he is fully conscious. Check to see if there are other injuries resulting from the fall.

Unless the fainting attack had an obvious cause, such as a fright, take your child to the doctor, even if he appears to be fully recovered.

Foreign bodies *see* Emergency Treatments, pages 42–3

Hiccups

Hiccups usually only last a few minutes. They are caused by involuntary contractions of the diaphragm and are not serious unless they last for two or three hours, in which case you should see a doctor.

If you want to try and stop the hiccups, tell your child to hold his breath or give him a long drink. If the hiccups continue, place a paper bag over his face and nose and tell your child to breathe in and out. **Never** use a plastic bag.

Newborn babies hiccup quite a lot and this is no cause for worry – it's a sign that the muscles involved in breathing are getting stronger and trying to work together.

Insect bites and stings

If your child is stung by a wasp, bee or hornet, it will be painful and frightening, but rarely dangerous.

A sting in the mouth or throat should be treated as urgent – the throat could swell very quickly making breathing difficult or impossible. To reduce the swelling, give him sips of iced water and get him to a hospital or doctor as soon as possible. If breathing becomes difficult place him in the recovery position (see page 20) and be ready to give mouth-to-mouth ventilation (see pages 16–17).

If your child is unduly sensitive to stings or is stung by, for example, a swarm of bees, he could develop anaphylactic shock (see page 24). To treat a sting that is not in the mouth or throat, gently pull the sting out with some tweezers if it is embedded in the skin. Avoid squeezing any poison sac that may be at the end of the sting as this could force the remaining poison into the skin. The area round the sting will be swollen, with a reddened point where the sting went in. Apply a cold compress to reduce the pain and swelling (see page 54) and antihistamine cream. The irritation usually fades in an hour or so, but see a doctor if it remains or increases in the next few days.

Jellyfish stings

Most jellyfish stings simply cause irritation although a few can be fatal. Tell your child to keep out of the way of jellyfish if he comes across them while swimming.

Wash jellyfish stings with sea water and put calamine lotion on the area that has been stung. Consult a doctor if the pain or swelling does not go within a couple of days.

Nosebleeds

This is usually due to bleeding from the blood vessels inside the nostrils.

Nosebleeds can be started by a blow to your child's nose or by him sneezing, picking or blowing his nose. If straw-coloured, blood-stained fluid rather than bright red blood is coming from his nose, this may be a sign of a fractured skull (see page 48), which requires urgent medical attention.

There can be a lot of blood with a nosebleed. If your child swallows or inhales this, it may cause vomiting or affect his breathing.

To treat the nosebleed, sit your child on your knee with his head well forward over a bowl, and loosen any tight clothing round his neck and chest. Using your finger and thumb, pinch the soft part of his nose for at least ten minutes, encouraging him to breathe through his mouth. Try and stop him talking or crying – the sooner he stops crying, the sooner the bleeding will stop.

Remove your finger and thumb after ten minutes; if the bleeding has not stopped, apply pressure for a further ten minutes. Don't let your child raise his head. When the bleeding has stopped, clean round the end of his nose with lukewarm water. Don't let your child run around or blow his nose for at least four hours after the bleeding stops.

If the bleeding has not stopped after thirty minutes, take your child to the doctor.

Your child may want to touch his nose while it is bleeding as it may feel numb, especially if the bleeding was started by a knock, and he may want to check it's still there. It's all right to let him do this so long as he does it gently.

Skin caught in a zip

If your child's skin gets caught in a zip, don't try to move the zip yourself; you will only make the injury worse and cause your child even more intense pain. Take your child to a hospital casualty department as quickly as possible. A cold compress (see page 54) placed over the zip will help relieve the pain in the meantime – you could also give him some junior paracetamol.

The hospital will inject a local anaesthetic, to numb the area round the zip, and then undo the zip.

Snake bites

Snake bites are rare in the UK; the only poisonous snake native to this country is the adder. In some countries there are numerous dangerous snakes and if your child is bitten while abroad, try and remember what the snake looked like (if you saw it) so it can be accurately identified.

If your child has been bitten by a snake, he may develop shock (see page 23) as a result of the fright, so you should treat this as well as the actual bite. Keep your child calm and still, and **don't** raise the bitten part above the level of his heart.

You will see one or two small puncture marks and some swelling where your child was bitten.

Clean the area round the bite and cover with a sterile dressing. If the bite is on an arm or leg, immobilize it by putting the arm in a sling (see page 57) or by bandaging one leg to the other as for a fracture (see page 46). Carry your child to the car or ambulance and take him to hospital.

Splinters

Splinters are small pieces of wood, glass or metal which can easily become embedded in the skin and may cause infection. Your child will probably complain of pain where the splinter has entered the skin.

Clean the area round the splinter, using cotton wool, soap and water. Then sterilize a pair of tweezers by passing them through a flame; allow them to cool, but don't wipe the soot off or touch the ends. Holding the tweezers as near to your child's skin as possible, grasp the end of the splinter and pull it out.

If the splinter breaks or you can't grasp the end, take your child to the doctor. **Never** dig into the skin to get at a splinter – you could push it further in. Check that your child's tetanus protection is up to date.

Sprains

Sprains usually happen to ankles and wrists and can be very painful.

Sometimes it can be difficult to tell if the injury is a sprain or a fracture and if you are in any doubt, treat it as a fracture (see pages 44–7). As well as pain, there will also probably be bruising and swelling and your child may not be able to move the injured joint.

Sit your child down and raise the injured part. A cold compress (see page 54) will help relieve pain and reduce swelling. With a sprained ankle, cover with a thick layer of cotton wool and bandage with a roller bandage (see page 55). A sprained wrist should be supported in an arm sling (see page 57). Take your child to the doctor.

Strains
Muscles can be strained by a sudden violent contraction or awkward movement. Your child will feel a sudden sharp pain and/or tenderness around the injured muscle and this may develop into stiffness or cramp. There may also be some swelling and discoloration.

As with a sprain, if you are in any doubt about the nature of the injury, treat it as a fracture (see pages 44–7).

Rest the injured part and reduce swelling by applying a cold compress (see page 54). Cover the muscle with a thick layer of cotton wool and bandage it firmly, but not too tightly, to counteract swelling. Raise the affected area. Take your child to a doctor if the injury seems severe.

Sunburn
Sunburn causes redness, itching and pain; in severe cases, blisters may form. You should always take great care to protect your child's skin from the sun. Introduce babies and young children to sunshine gradually – for five to ten minutes on the first day, increasing it little by little each day thereafter. Use a high protection factor sunscreen cream on any exposed areas of their skin and reapply it every few hours or after they have been in the water. Always use a sunshade for a baby and put the pram or pushchair where there is

a slight breeze. Give children lots to drink in hot weather.

In strong sun, make your child wear a T-shirt, shorts and a hat, even when he's swimming.

Remember that sunburn can also happen on cloudy days in summer and as a result of the reflection of the sun's rays on snow.

If your child does get sunburn, move him to the shade and sponge his skin with tepid water to cool it. Give him sips of cold water. Calamine lotion will help to cool the skin or you can use special after-sun creams. Giving junior paracetamol will also help relieve any soreness.

If the sunburn is severe or your child develops a high temperature, you should call the doctor; a high temperature may indicate heatstroke (see page 49).

Tooth injury see Bleeding tooth socket

USEFUL ADDRESSES

British Red Cross Society
9 Grosvenor Crescent
London SW1X 7EJ
(01) 235 5454

St John Ambulance
1 Grosvenor Crescent
London SW1X 7EF
(01) 235 5231

St Andrew's Ambulance Association
St Andrew's House
48 Milton Street
Glasgow G4 0HR
(041) 332 4031

Royal Life Saving Society UK
Mounbatten House
Studley
Warwickshire B80 7NN
(052785) 3943

Child Accident Prevention Trust
75 Portland Place
London W1N 3AL
(01) 636 2545

INDEX